CNA

Study Guide

2023-2024 Edition

Ace the Certified Nursing Assistant Exam on Your First Try with No Effort | Test Questions, Answer Keys & Tips to Score a 98% Pass Rate

GERALD SACKLER

Table of Contents

INTRODUCTION _____ **9**

CHAPTER 1: THE CNA EXAM _____ **11**

IMPORTANCE OF THE CNA EXAM _____ 11

ELIGIBILITY REQUIREMENTS _____ 12

    Age Requirements _____ 12

    Education and Training Prerequisites _____ 12

    Criminal Background Check _____ 13

    Immunization and Health Requirements _____ 13

    State-specific Requirements _____ 14

HOW TO REGISTER FOR THE EXAM? _____ 14

    Researching Approved Testing Agencies _____ 14

    Application Process _____ 15

    Required Documents and Fees _____ 15

PREPARING FOR THE EXAM _____ 15

    Scheduling the Exam Date _____ 16

    Recommended Study Materials _____ 16

    Reviewing Course Content _____ 17

    Practice Tests and Mock Exams _____ 17

    Seeking Additional Resources (e.g., textbooks, online resources) ____ 17

EXAM FORMAT AND CONTENT _____ 18

    Written (Knowledge) Exam _____ 18

    Number of Questions _____ 19

    Time Limit _____ 19

    Content Areas (e.g., basic nursing skills, infection control, safety measures) ____ 20

    Clinical Skills Exam _____ 20

    Purpose and Format _____ 21

    Required Skills to Demonstrate _____ 21

    Evaluation Criteria _____ 21

EXAM DAY _____ 22

Preparing in Advance _____ 22

Arriving at the Testing Center _____ 23

Arriving at the Testing Center _____ 23

Written Exam _____ 24

Clinical Skills Exam _____ 24

Post-Exam Procedures _____ 24

CHAPTER 2: HOW TO PASS THE CNA EXAM? _____ 27

IMPORTANCE OF PASSING THE CNA EXAM _____ 27

TEST PREPARATION _____ 28

Create a study plan _____ 28

Gather study materials _____ 28

STUDY STRATEGY _____ 29

Create a study schedule _____ 29

Utilize different study methods _____ 30

Seek additional resources or support _____ 30

TEST-TAKING TIPS _____ 30

Manage your time effectively_____ 31

Answer confidently but avoid guessing _____ 31

REVIEW YOUR ANSWERS _____ 32

OVERCOMING TEST ANXIETY _____ 32

Understand the causes of test anxiety_____ 33

PRACTICE RELAXATION TECHNIQUES_____ 34

Develop a positive mindset _____ 34

CHAPTER 3: PHYSICAL CARE SKILLS _____ 37

THE IMPORTANCE OF PHYSICAL CARE SKILLS _____ 37

THE CNA EXAM AND PHYSICAL CARE SKILLS _____ 38

PERSONAL CARE _____ 38

DRESSING AND GROOMING _____ 39

NUTRITION AND HYDRATION _____ 39

RESTORATION AND MAINTENANCE OF HEALTH _____ 40

SLEEP AND REST NEEDS _____ 40

ELIMINATION (BOWEL AND BLADDER)_____ 41

MOBILITY, INCLUDING IMPAIRED MOBILITY _____ 41

CIRCULATION AND SKIN INTEGRITY_____ 42

ELIMINATION (BLADDER AND BOWEL)_____ 42

PATTERNS OF SLEEP AND REST 43

SELF-IMAGE 43

STRENGTH AND ENDURANCE 44

CARE AND USE OF ASSISTIVE DEVICES 44

AGE-RELATED CHANGES 45

COGNITIVE CHANGES 45

PSYCHOSOCIAL CHANGES 46

PHYSICAL CHANGES 47

PSYCHOSOCIAL NEEDS 47

CHAPTER 4: NURSING CARE 49

DUTIES OF A CNA 49

IMPORTANCE OF OBSERVATION AND REPORTING IN NURSING CARE 50

OBSERVATION AND REPORTING PHYSICAL CHANGES 50

Definition and importance of physical changes 51

Techniques for observing physical changes 51

Reporting methods and documentation 52

Case studies and practice scenarios 52

BASIC ANATOMY AND FUNCTIONS OF BODY SYSTEMS 53

Overview of major body systems 53

Anatomy and functions of each body system 54

Characteristics of Body Functions 54

Normal body functions and vital signs 54

Abnormal body functions and signs of illness 55

Assessing and monitoring body functions 55

Recognizing and reporting changes in body functions 56

Observation and Reporting of Behavior Changes 56

Understanding behavior changes in patients 57

Techniques for observing and documenting behavior changes 57

CHANGES IN MENTAL STATUS (CONFUSION) 58

Definition and causes of mental status changes 58

Signs and symptoms of Confusion 59

Techniques for assessing and monitoring mental status 59

ORIENTATION/VALIDATION TECHNIQUES 60

Importance of orientation and validation in patient care 60

Techniques for orienting and validating patients 60

Strategies for providing a supportive environment 61

Case studies and role-playing exercises 61

EMOTIONAL STRESS _____ 62

    Understanding emotional stress and its impact on patients _____ 62

MOOD STATUS CHANGES _____ 62

    A. Definition and Causes of Mood Status Changes: _____ 62

    B. Assessing and Monitoring Mood Status: _____ 63

    C. Techniques for Promoting Positive Mood and Emotional Well-being: ____ 64

DEFENSE MECHANISMS _____ 64

    A. Overview of Defense Mechanisms in Psychology: _____ 64

    B. Recognizing and Understanding Common Defense Mechanisms: _____ 64

    C. Interactions between Defense Mechanisms and Patient Care: _____ 65

ACUTE EMERGENCIES _____ 65

CHAPTER 5: SPECIALIZED CARE _____ 67

INTRODUCTION TO SPECIALIZED CARE _____ 67

    Importance of specialized care for patients with physical and psychological problems _____ 67

    Role of the CNA in providing specialized care _____ 68

    Physical Problems _____ 68

    Understanding physical impairments _____ 69

    Providing for patient safety _____ 69

    Care and comfort for patients with physical impairments _____ 70

    Psychological Problems _____ 70

    Understanding psychological problems _____ 71

    Care of the Dying Patient _____ 71

POSTMORTEM CARE _____ 72

CHAPTER 6: THE ROLE OF THE CNA (ROLE OF THE NURSE AID) __ 75

WHAT DOES A CNA DO? _____ 75

THE IMPORTANCE OF THE CNA ROLE _____ 76

PERSONAL RESPONSIBILITY _____ 76

PERSONAL HEALTH AND SAFETY _____ 77

DISPOSAL OF POINTED OR SHARP OBJECTS _____ 77

PATIENT RIGHTS _____ 78

LEGAL BEHAVIOR _____ 78

ETHICAL BEHAVIOR _____ 79

PRIORITIZATION AND TIME MANAGEMENT _____ 79

PRINCIPLES OF TEAMWORK _____ 80

INTERPERSONAL RELATIONS AND COMMUNICATION SKILLS IN HEALTH CARE _____ 80

Therapeutic communication techniques _____ 81

CHAPTER 7: QUESTIONS _____ 83

CHAPTER 8: ANSWERS & EXPLANATION _____ 99

CONCLUSION_____ 107

Introduction

It is the dream of many people to pass the CNA exam. So, becoming a Certified Nursing Assistant (CNA) is a career choice and a calling for those passionate about helping others and providing compassionate care. CNAs are the backbone of healthcare, working alongside nurses and healthcare professionals to ensure patients receive the highest respect and support.

The CNA Exam is a crucial step to becoming a certified professional. This comprehensive assessment evaluates your knowledge, skills, and abilities in patient care, including vital signs monitoring, personal hygiene assistance, e.g., variance, mobility support, and effective communication.

Excelling in the CNA Exam is more than just passing a test; it's about developing a solid foundation of knowledge and honing essential skills that will serve you throughout your career. This comprehensive guide crafts to provide you with the tools, strategies, and resources needed to navigate the challenges of the CNA Exam with confidence and competence.

This book will give you a wealth of information and guidance to help you prepare effectively for the CNA Exam. We begin by exploring the importance of CNA certification and the numerous opportunities and rewards that come with it. Understanding this exam's significance and role in your professional journey will motivate and inspire you to strive for excellence.

To help you succeed in the CNA Exam, we have included detailed chapters covering each examination component. You will discover valuable tips and techniques to optimize your study habits, create a personalized study plan, and maximize available resources. Whether you prefer textbooks, online courses, or practice exams, we provide recommendations. And guidance to ensure you have the right tools will.

The written component of the CNA Exam demands a solid understanding of theoretical knowledge in anatomy, physiology, medical terminology, and healthcare ethics. Our chapter dedicated to this section offers a comprehensive content review, sample questions, and strategies for effective time management during the exam.

In addition to the written component, the CNA Exam includes a practical skills assessment. We walk you through the essential skills and procedures you will be evaluated on, providing clear explanations, step-by-step instructions, and visual aids to enhance your learning experience. Practice scenarios and checklists will help you gain confidence in performing these skills accurately and efficiently.

Throughout the book, we emphasize the importance of critical thinking, professionalism, and effective communication, as these qualities are vital for success in the CNA Exam and your future career as a healthcare professional. We guide how to approach different types of questions, communicate effectively with patients and their families, and maintain professionalism in various healthcare settings.

As you embark on this journey to become a Certified Nursing Assistant, "CNA Study Guide" will be your trusted companion. With proper preparation, a positive mindset, and the knowledge and skills acquired through this book, you will confidently pass the CNA Exam and embark on a fulfilling career dedicated to caring for others.

Chapter 1

The CNA Exam

Are you considering a career as a Certified Nursing Assistant (CNA)? If so, it's important to know that passing the CNA exam is essential in becoming certified and starting your journey in the healthcare industry. However, with so many requirements and state-specific regulations to navigate, it can be overwhelming. That's why we are trying to make a comprehensive guide about the CNA exam. From age requirements and education prerequisites to researching approved testing agencies and scheduling your exam date – we've got you covered! So, let's start breaking down this crucial chapter of your CNA journey.

Importance of the CNA Exam

The CNA exam is critical to obtaining certification as a nursing assistant. The purpose is to test your knowledge and skills in caring for patients across various healthcare services, including hospitals, long-term care facilities, and home health agencies.

Passing the CNA exam means demonstrating competency in primary patient care, infection control measures, communication with patients and their families, safety protocols, and emergency procedures. As an essential healthcare worker, you must possess these fundamental skills to ensure safe and efficient patient care.

Moreover, becoming certified can open up many employment opportunities for CNAs across different states in the US. Many employers require certification as proof of competency before hiring nursing assistants. A CNA certification can also provide a steppingstone toward pursuing higher education or advancing within the field.

Passing the CNA exam is more than just about getting certified – it's about demonstrating what it takes to be an efficient caregiver who provides quality patient care while maintaining high ethical standards in your practice.

Eligibility Requirements

Familiarizing yourself with the eligibility requirements—the essential ones mentioned below is vital.

Age Requirements

Becoming a Certified Nursing Assistant (CNA) requires individuals to meet specific age requirements. The minimum age requirement for taking the CNA exam can change from state to state but usually ranges between 16 and 18 years old.

The objective is to ensure that CNAs are mature enough to care for patients. It also ensures they have completed a significant portion of their high school education and possess primary language and math skills.

While some states allow minors to take the exam with parental consent, others require all candidates to be legal adults before allowing them to test. Additionally, even if you can take the exam as a minor, it may limit your job opportunities since many healthcare facilities prefer employees over 18 years old.

Meeting age requirements is an essential step towards becoming a CNA. Make sure you research your state's specific regulations regarding minimum age so you can plan accordingly.

Education and Training Prerequisites

Before taking the Certified Nursing Assistant (CNA) exam, it is essential to meet all educational and training prerequisites. While these requirements may vary depending on the state, specific universal qualifications exist.

Candidates must hold a high school diploma or GED equivalent before enrolling in a CNA program. Additionally, applicants should have basic knowledge of math and reading comprehension skills to understand medical terminologies accurately.

CNA programs typically last between four and twelve weeks. During this time frame, students will learn fundamental nursing skills such as bathing patients, changing bed linens, monitoring vital signs, and administering medication.

The courses will also cover safety procedures for patients and healthcare workers to reduce accidents or injuries in a hospital setting.

In classroom instruction, students will receive hands-on training through clinical rotations at local healthcare facilities. This practical experience allows aspiring CNAs to apply their newly acquired skills under professional supervision.

Meeting all educational and training prerequisites required by your state's Board of Nursing before taking the CNA exam can help you achieve success on test day!

Criminal Background Check

Before taking the CNA exam, candidates need to undergo a criminal background check. It is to ensure that the individuals working with vulnerable populations such as seniors and disabled individuals have no prior criminal records.

The criminal background check typically involves a fingerprinting process to investigate an individual's records thoroughly. Candidates must disclose any previous convictions or pending charges during their application process, as failure to do so may result in disqualification from taking the exam.

It is worth noting that having a prior conviction does not automatically disqualify someone from becoming a certified nursing assistant. However, some severe offenses, such as those related to abuse, neglect, or exploitation of vulnerable persons, may bar someone from being eligible for certification.

Candidates should also comply with all state-specific background checks and disclosure requirements. Being transparent about one's history can increase trustworthiness and credibility when applying for jobs after passing the CNA exam.

Immunization and Health Requirements

As a prospective Certified Nursing Assistant (CNA), meeting specific health prerequisites before taking the CNA exam is crucial. These requirements are in place to ensure the safety of both healthcare workers and patients under their care.

In most states, immunizations play a significant role in fulfilling these health prerequisites. CNAs need to be up-to-date on vaccines such as Hepatitis B, MMR (measles, mumps, and rubella), Tdap (tetanus, diphtheria, pertussis), varicella (chickenpox), and an annual flu shot. Some states or testing centers may have additional vaccination requirements.

Apart from immunizations, applicants must also provide proof of negative TB tests within the past 12 months; in some cases where further evaluation is needed – like when there's a history of positive TB test results – a chest X-ray might require.

Potential CNAs should undergo general physical exams with documentation stating they're physically fit for nursing work. It may include assessing one's weightlifting abilities or checking for any underlying medical conditions affecting job performance.

Meeting these immunization and health requirements before your CNA exam application process ensures you are well-prepared for the examination and your future career in healthcare!

State-specific Requirements

Each state has its unique requirements when it comes to the CNA exam. Researching and understanding these requirements before beginning the application process is essential.

Some states may require additional training or education beyond the federal minimum, while others may have different age or health requirement standards.

For example, in California, candidates must complete a 150-hour training program approved by the state's Department of Public Health. In Texas, candidates must pass a competency evaluation program, including written and skills tests.

It is crucial to carefully review each state's specific requirements as they can vary significantly from one another. It will ensure that you are fully prepared for your exam and meet all necessary qualifications.

Additionally, some states may require CNAs to complete continuing education courses to maintain their certification. It is essential to stay up-to-date with any changes or updates in your state's regulations regarding CNAs.

How to Register for the Exam?

Once you get all the necessary and relevant details about the exam, the next step is to register.

Researching Approved Testing Agencies

The CNA exam is a crucial step toward becoming a certified nursing assistant. One important aspect that you need to consider before taking the test is researching approved testing agencies.

Each state has a list of approved testing agencies; choosing one that meets your requirements is essential. You can find the list on your state's Department of Health website or by contacting them directly.

When researching, make sure to check the agency's reputation and credibility. Look for reviews from previous examinees and ask around among healthcare professionals.

It's also essential to consider location and scheduling options when choosing an agency. Choose an agency near you for convenience so you don't have to travel far on exam day.

Check if the agency offers additional resources, such as study materials or practice tests, which could help you better prepare for the exam.

Researching approved testing agencies is crucial in preparing for the CNA exam. Choosing an agency that fits your needs will relax you during this hectic process.

Application Process

The application process for the CNA exam is relatively straightforward but can be time-consuming. Before starting your application, ensure that you have met all the prerequisites specific to your state.

To begin, obtain an application form from a testing agency approved by your state's regulatory body. Fill out the form completely and provide accurate information about yourself and any required documentation, such as proof of education or immunization records.

Next, submit the completed application and any necessary fees to the appropriate agency. The CNA exam cost varies depending on location but typically ranges between $50-$200.

When your application is submitted, reviewed, and processed, you will receive confirmation of eligibility for the exam. It may include instructions on scheduling a test date at a designated facility in your area.

It is vital to note that some states require applicants to apply directly through their state's regulatory body rather than through third-party testing agencies. Be sure to research state-specific requirements before beginning your application process.

While applying for the CNA exam may seem overwhelming at first glance, it is a necessary step towards achieving certification as a nursing assistant and advancing in this rewarding career field.

Required Documents and Fees

Before scheduling your CNA exam, you must have all the necessary documents. These typically include a government-issued ID, proof of high school or GED completion, and completed training program hours documentation.

Additionally, the fee associated with taking the CNA exam varies by state. The cost can range from $50 to 200 dollars, and you must pay before scheduling your exam date. Some conditions may also require additional fees for fingerprinting and background checks.

It's essential to note that some states may have different requirements in terms of documentation and fees, so it's crucial to check with your state's nursing board for specific information.

Gather all required documents and pay any necessary fees before your desired exam date. It will ensure a smooth process when registering for the test without any last-minute surprises or complications!

Preparing for the Exam

Preparing for the CNA Exam is crucial to ensure success and confidence on the examination day. It involves studying the necessary knowledge and practicing the required clinical skills. By understanding the exam format and content, gathering appropriate study materials, and utilizing practice resources, candidates can effectively prepare themselves.

Scheduling the Exam Date

After preparing for the CNA exam, the next step is to schedule a date to take the test. Choosing a time when you feel most confident and prepared is essential. The scheduling process can vary depending on your state's requirements.

Most states allow candidates to register online through their website or by phone. You will need personal information like name, address, social security number, and payment details like credit card information. Ensure to have all the required documents ready before starting registration.

When choosing a date for your exam, consider how much time you need to prepare adequately. It's best to take the test before it because knowledge retention decreases over time.

Ensure you understand any fees associated with rescheduling or canceling an exam if unforeseen events make it impossible to sit for the scheduled date.

Scheduling your CNA exam requires careful planning and consideration of various factors such as availability and preparation level. Take your time during this process to fully prepare on testing day!

Recommended Study Materials

Preparing for the CNA exam can be daunting but much more manageable with suitable study materials. Here are some recommended study materials that will help you ace the exam.

First and foremost, consider purchasing an official CNA Exam Prep book. These books are explicitly tailored to the exam's content and provide valuable insights into what to expect on test day. They also often come with practice exams and sample questions.

Invest in flashcards covering key terms and concepts commonly found on the exam. Flashcards offer a convenient way to review information quickly during free moments throughout your day.

Another helpful resource is online courses or tutorials. Many websites offer video lessons that cover essential topics tested on the CNA exam in-depth. It is beneficial for visual learners who benefit from seeing demonstrations of specific skills, such as transferring patients or taking vital signs.

Remember to consider the value of practicing with mock exams! Many official prep books have these tests included to assess how well you're doing before test day arrives.

In summary, having access to quality study materials is an integral part of preparing for success on any standardized test, including The Certified Nursing Assistant (CNA) Exam.

Reviewing Course Content

Reviewing course content is one of the most crucial steps in preparing for the CNA exam. It's essential to ensure you understand all the material in your training program, as this will test on the exam.

To begin with, take a look at your course syllabus or outline and identify topics that may require additional review. It could include basic nursing skills such as taking vital signs or assisting with daily living activities, infection control measures, safety precautions, etc.

Consider creating flashcards or study guides to help you memorize key terms and concepts related to each topic area. You can use many online resources, such as educational videos or interactive quizzes, to reinforce your understanding of specific subjects.

It's essential not just to memorize information but also to apply it in practical scenarios. Consider practicing procedures like handwashing techniques or changing bed linens so that you feel confident in your abilities when it comes time for the clinical portion of the exam.

By thoroughly reviewing course content and applying it practically, you'll equip for success on the CNA exam.

Practice Tests and Mock Exams

Practice tests and mock exams are essential to prepare for the CNA exam. These practice tests can help you gain familiarity with the types of questions that will ask on the actual exam, as well as identify areas where you may need more study.

Taking multiple practice tests from different sources is essential to comprehensively understanding the material. Mock exams can also help simulate test-taking conditions and provide an opportunity to assess your readiness for the exam.

One recommended resource for practice tests is the official CNA Exam Prep app, which includes over 700 questions and detailed explanations. Other options include online resources such as Quizlet or purchasing study guides with practice test materials.

Simulating testing conditions when taking practice tests is vital by setting aside uninterrupted time and using only approved reference materials. It helps build confidence, reduce anxiety during testing, and ultimately leads to better performance on test day.

Incorporating regular practice tests into your study routine effectively increases your chances of passing the CNA exam on your first attempt.

Seeking Additional Resources (e.g., textbooks, online resources)

As you prepare for the CNA exam, you must have many resources. While reviewing your course content and taking practice tests are essential to your preparation, seeking additional materials can help solidify your knowledge and boost your confidence.

One excellent resource is textbooks specifically designed for preparing for the CNA exam. These books often provide in-depth explanations of key concepts and include practice questions that closely resemble those on the test. Look for reputable publishers who have experience creating study materials for nursing exams.

Another option is online resources such as forums, blogs, and videos. These can offer valuable insights from other students who have taken the exam or from instructors with expertise in CNA training. Many websites offer free or low-cost practice tests and flashcards to help you review important information quickly.

It's also worth considering joining a study group or finding a tutor if you need more personalized assistance. It allows you to ask questions tailored to your learning style while benefitting from others' experiences.

Remember that while these additional resources can be helpful, they should not replace dedicated studying using official course materials approved by testing organizations. Use them as supplements rather than primary sources of information so that you cover all necessary topics comprehensively!

Exam Format and Content

The CNA exam consists of written (knowledge) and clinical skills exams. The written exam typically includes multiple-choice questions assessing various nursing knowledge areas, such as basic skills, safety measures, and infection control. The clinical skills exam evaluates the candidate's ability to perform essential nursing tasks, such as taking vital signs, assisting with personal care, and maintaining a safe environment. It is necessary for candidates to thoroughly understand the format and content of both exams to prepare and succeed effectively.

Written (Knowledge) Exam

The written (knowledge) exam is crucial to the CNA certification process. This test assesses your understanding of basic nursing skills, infection control, safety measures, and other content areas relevant to the profession.

Before taking the exam, make sure you have thoroughly reviewed all the course materials and practice tests. The more prepared you are for this exam, the higher your chances of passing it on your first try.

During the test itself, be sure to read each question carefully before selecting an answer. Pace yourself throughout the exam to have enough time to complete all questions within the allotted time limit.

Remember that passing this exam is essential in obtaining your CNA certification. Therefore, taking this portion seriously and giving it ample attention during preparation is vital.

You can pass this knowledge-based examination with flying colors by being well-prepared and confident during testing!

Number of Questions

One of the vital aspects of preparing for the CNA exam is understanding what to expect on test day. It includes knowing how many questions you must answer during the written (knowledge) exam.

The number of questions on the CNA exam can vary by state but generally ranges from 70-100 multiple-choice questions. It's important to note that not all questions carry equal weight; some may be pre-test or experimental items that are not scored.

It would help if you manage your time so that you have enough time to answer each question thoroughly; I recommend that you consume one minute on each question. If you spend too much time on a question, mark it for review and move on to save time before answering every question.

Notably, some states may require an additional skills evaluation in addition to the written portion of the exam. The skills evaluation typically involves performing five randomly selected nursing assistant duties before a proctor who will evaluate your performance.

By familiarizing yourself with the number and format of questions ahead of time and practicing efficient test-taking strategies like pacing yourself, you'll be better prepared for a successful test day.

Time Limit

The CNA exam is a timed test with two parts: a written multiple-choice test and a clinical skills examination. The duration of the written portion of the exam differs state by state but typically ranges from 90 minutes to two hours. You'll need to answer anywhere from 60 to 100 questions during this time.

It's essential to manage your time wisely during the written test. Reading each question carefully and spending little time on any question is necessary. If you need help with an answer, skip it and return if time remains.

The clinical skills examination also has a time limit that varies by state but usually lasts 30-40 minutes per candidate. During this part of the exam, you'll ask to perform five randomly selected nursing skills in front of an evaluator.

To ensure you complete all required tasks within the given timeframe, practice performing each skill efficiently before taking your exam. Time yourself while practicing to get used to working under pressure and make adjustments as needed.

Remember - managing your time is crucial when taking the CNA exam!

Content Areas (e.g., basic nursing skills, infection control, safety measures)

The Certified Nursing Assistant (CNA) exam is a comprehensive assessment that evaluates your ability to provide primary nursing care. The exam's content areas are needed to assess your knowledge and skills in each aspect of patient care.

Basic nursing skills are one of the primary content areas covered in the CNA exam. This area includes bathing, grooming, feeding, and assisting with mobility. You will expect to demonstrate proficiency in these fundamental skills during the test's written and clinical portions.

Another critical area evaluated on the CNA exam is infection control. As a healthcare professional, it's essential to understand how infections spread and how to prevent their transmission effectively. You'll need to know about proper hand hygiene techniques, standard precautions for preventing infection, and recognizing signs of infectious disease.

Safety measures are also an essential consideration in the CNA exam. This category covers fall prevention strategies, safe patient handling techniques, fire safety protocols, and emergency preparedness procedures.

You must have a solid understanding of each content area before taking the CNA exam to perform well on both written questions and clinical evaluations related to those subjects. By mastering these key concepts beforehand through study materials or review sessions with other CNAs-in-training or working professionals alike - you can feel more confident going into the testing day!

Clinical Skills Exam

The Clinical Skills Exam is the practical portion of the CNA exam, where test takers demonstrate their ability to perform essential nursing skills. This exam portion typically occurs in a simulated clinical setting, with actors playing patients for the test taker to interact with.

During this part of the exam, candidates will ask to demonstrate five randomly selected skills from a list provided by their state's board of nursing. These skills may include taking vital signs, bathing patients, and transferring them from bed to wheelchair.

It's essential for candidates to thoroughly review all potential skills on their state's list ahead of time and practice performing them in a simulated environment. It will help ensure they feel confident and prepared when it comes time for the actual exam.

In addition to technical proficiency in these tasks, candidates must also display strong communication skills and an ability to provide compassionate care throughout each scenario presented during the Clinical Skills Exam.

Purpose and Format

The CNA exam aims to evaluate that candidates must have the required knowledge and skills to provide quality care to patients in a healthcare setting. This exam divides into two parts: a written examination and a clinical skills examination.

The written portion assesses the candidate's understanding of basic nursing skills, infection control, safety measures, communication, and patient rights. It comprises multiple-choice questions that test knowledge retention and application abilities.

On the other hand, the clinical skills portion evaluates how well candidates can perform specific tasks while following proper procedures. This part requires candidates to demonstrate proficiency in five randomly selected nursing assistant duties within thirty minutes.

Candidates must have an excellent grasp of theoretical concepts and practical applications. Additionally, they must manage their time effectively during both parts of the examination.

Understanding its purpose and format helps aspiring CNAs prepare adequately for success in this critical evaluation.

Required Skills to Demonstrate

You must demonstrate various skills essential to providing quality patient care to pass the CNA exam. These skills divide into two categories: cognitive and psychomotor.

Cognitive skills refer to your ability to understand and recall vital information related to patient care, such as identifying different types of medication or recognizing signs of infection. To succeed in this area, you must diligently study and dedicate daily time to reviewing the material.

Psychomotor skills, on the other hand, involve applying what you have learned in a hands-on setting. It includes tasks like measuring vital signs or assisting with activities of daily living (ADLs). You will need to practice these skills extensively before taking the exam so that they become second nature.

In addition to technical abilities, CNAs must also display strong communication and interpersonal skills when working with patients. It involves listening attentively, empathizing with their concerns, and communicating effectively with healthcare professionals.

Passing the CNA exam requires knowledge and practical experience that can only come from putting in hard work through study sessions and training programs.

Evaluation Criteria

Evaluation criteria are the standards by which your performance on the CNA exam will measure. These criteria determine whether or not you pass the exam and receive your certification. Paying to these evaluation criteria when preparing for your test is essential.

Your performance on written and clinical skills exams will evaluate basis on a set of predetermined guidelines. For example, in the clinical skills portion, candidates must demonstrate competency in hand washing, measuring vital signs, and assisting with patient mobility. Each task asses using a specific checklist that provides detailed instructions on performing each skill correctly.

In addition to performing tasks correctly, candidates must demonstrate professional behavior during their examination. It includes displaying good communication skills with patients and staff members, maintaining appropriate boundaries during procedures, and protecting patient privacy and dignity at all times.

While there is no single key factor determining success or failure on the CNA exam, understanding what evaluation criteria involve can significantly increase your chances of passing this challenging assessment. By studying carefully beforehand and paying close attention to detail when carrying out tasks throughout the testing day, you'll improve your probability of becoming certified as a nursing assistant!

Exam Day

On the day of the CNA exam, arriving at the testing center on time is crucial, allowing for any necessary travel or unforeseen delays. Candidates should ensure they have all the required documents, such as identification and registration confirmation, to facilitate a smooth check-in process. Adhering to the appropriate dress code, which typically includes wearing scrubs or professional attire, demonstrates professionalism and respect for the exam environment. It is also essential to bring any necessary supplies, such as a watch for timekeeping and comfortable, non-slip shoes for the clinical skills portion of the exam.

Preparing in Advance

The Certified Nursing Assistant (CNA) exam can be a hectic experience, but you can increase your chances of success with proper preparation. Here are practical steps on how to prepare for the exam:

Firstly, review the content areas covered in the exam, such as basic nursing skills, infection control, and safety measures. You can find study guides online or invest in a reputable review book.

Next, take practice tests to familiarize yourself with the questions you'll encounter and develop test-taking strategies. It will help reduce anxiety during the actual exam.

In addition to reviewing written material, practicing clinical skills is also essential. Work through practical scenarios with a professional nurse or healthcare provider who can give you feedback on your technique.

Getting enough rest before the CNA exam is important since fatigue may affect performance negatively. On examination day, arrive early, at least thirty minutes before start time; this gives ample time for check-in procedures like ID verification and fingerprinting.

In summary, preparing well ahead of time by studying both theoretical materials and practical situations is crucial if one wants to pass their exams successfully!

Arriving at the Testing Center

Arriving at the testing center for the Certified Nursing Assistant (CNA) Exam can be nerve-wracking. You want to ensure you're on time, prepared, and in the right mindset. Here are some tips to help you perform well.

First, ensure you know where the testing center's location and how long it will take you to get there. Give yourself enough time to arrive at least 30 minutes before your exam.

Dress appropriately – business casual or scrubs recommend since this is a professional exam. Avoid wearing anything too flashy or distracting, as that may impact your concentration during the test.

Bring all required documents, such as identification and admission ticket. Double-check that everything is in order before leaving home.

Once at the testing center, take deep breaths and relax your mind. Use any wait time to review key terms or concepts that may appear on the exam.

Remember that nerves are normal, but don't let them overshadow your hard work preparing for this momentous occasion! Stay positive, focused, and confident, knowing that you have put forth diligent effort toward achieving success on test day!

Arriving at the Testing Center

Arriving at the testing center can be nerve-wracking, but staying calm and focused is essential. It would help if you reached early enough for any unexpected delays on your journey. Rushing into the test center gives rise to stress that can negatively affect your performance during the exam.

Upon arrival, check in with the official at the reception desk, who will confirm your registration details before directing you towards a waiting area where you'll wait until called upon by an invigilator or examiner.

Before entering the examination hall, ensure that all prohibited items, such as phones and bags, are left outside or in designated lockers provided by the testing center. The CNA Exam monitor strictly, so do not bring anything other than acceptable identification documents.

Take deep breaths and exhale while visualizing yourself passing this crucial stage of becoming a certified nursing assistant. Remembering these simple tips can help ease anxiety-related issues upon arriving at the testing center.

Written Exam

The written exam is one of the two parts of the CNA certification test. It consists of multiple-choice questions that evaluate your knowledge and understanding of various topics related to nursing care. Here are some notable tips to pass the written exam.

Firstly, make sure you understand the format and structure of the exam. The CNA exam usually has 60-70 multiple-choice questions, which must complete within two hours. You must read each question carefully before answering it, as some answers may seem correct at first glance but could be incorrect on closer inspection.

Secondly, take practice tests and review study materials regularly. It will help you familiarize yourself with common questions asked in the trial and improve your chances of passing with flying colors.

Remember to use time management skills when taking the test. Make sure you pace yourself wisely during those two hours and try not to waste too much time on any one question.

Success in this part comes from preparation, focus, and determination!

Clinical Skills Exam

The Clinical Skills Exam is the second part of the CNA exam. This section tests your ability to perform various nursing procedures on a patient in a simulated clinical setting. The skills include taking vital signs, feeding patients, assisting with mobility, and other tasks that CNAs commonly perform.

Before beginning this exam section, you will get instructions on what tasks you need to complete for each scenario. You will then have a certain amount of time to complete each task while being observed by an examiner.

It's important to remember that during this portion of the exam, you must demonstrate proper technique and follow infection control protocols at all times. Make sure to wash your hands frequently and wear gloves when appropriate.

Practicing these skills with friends or family members who can act as patients is vital. This way, you'll feel more comfortable and confident regarding the test.

Remember that this portion of the CNA exam tests your ability to provide safe and effective care as a certified nursing assistant.

Post-Exam Procedures

After taking the Certified Nursing need constant (CNA) exam, you must know what is next. Well, there are a few things that you need to remember when it comes to post-exam procedures.

Firstly, collect your belongings before leaving the testing center after your exam. It's also important to take some time and relax after such an intense experience.

Next up is waiting for your results. Depending on state regulations, you may receive immediate feedback or wait a few weeks for your official scores. In either case, try not to stress too much and focus on other things while waiting.

Once you receive your scores and find out that you've passed the CNA exam, congratulations! You're now eligible for certification and can start applying for jobs as a CNA. However, if unfortunately didn't pass this time around, don't worry about it- use this experience as motivation towards future success!

Remember that becoming a CNA is an accomplishment worth celebrating regardless of whether or not you passed on the first try and keep pushing forward towards achieving further success in the healthcare industry!

Becoming a Certified Nursing Assistant is no easy feat, and passing the CNA exam is essential in beginning your healthcare professional career. With proper preparation and dedication, you can confidently approach the test and successfully pass both the written and clinical skills portions.

Ensure you reach the testing center early to have enough time to check in and settle before starting your exam. During the written portion of the test, take your time reading each question carefully to make your final decision. Take your time completing your paper. Take your time and solve it wisely.

For the clinical skills exam, practicing beforehand can help you feel more comfortable performing in front of an evaluator. You may utilize the resources like online tutorials or hands-on training sessions offered by nursing schools or local healthcare organizations.

After completing both sections of the CNA exam, follow all post-exam procedures provided by your state's nursing board. It may include waiting for official results or submitting additional documentation for certification purposes.

Passing the CNA exam requires hard work and dedication, but achieving this milestone will open up many opportunities within healthcare. By following these tips and consistently studying and practicing for exams, you, too, can become a successful certified nursing assistant.

Chapter 2

How To Pass The CNA Exam?

Are you super excited to have a promising career in nursing? Getting a Certified Nursing Assistant (CNA) into the healthcare industry is an excellent choice. However, before you can start caring for patients and making a difference in their lives, there's one hurdle that you need to overcome - passing the CNA exam. Don't worry; it may seem daunting at first, but with proper preparation and study strategies, you'll pass with flying colors! This chapter guides you through HOW TO PASS THE CNA EXAM successfully. So, let's get started!

Importance of passing the CNA exam

Becoming a CNA is an admirable and rewarding career choice. In a CNA career, you will be responsible and in charge of providing direct patient care under the supervision of licensed nurses. It is a must for you to become certified; you have to pass the CNA exam.

The importance of passing this test cannot overstate. It demonstrates your competence and knowledge in providing patient care and ensures that you meet the state-specific requirements for employment as a nursing assistant.

Furthermore, passing the CNA exam opens up opportunities for career advancement in healthcare. Many CNAs pursue further education or training programs such as Licensed Practical Nurse (LPN) or Registered Nurse (RN).

Passing the CNA exam is vital for obtaining certification and advancing your career in healthcare while positively impacting patients' lives.

Test Preparation

Preparing for any exam requires dedication, planning, and effort. The Certified Nursing Assistant (CNA) Exam is no different. Aspiring CNAs who want to pass the CNA Exam must develop a solid test preparation strategy. It is not an easy exam, so you require proper planning and execution of your planning. You have to make up a plan and stick to it. Consistency can take you toward success. Here are some fantastic tips which will guide you to pass this exam.

Create a study plan

Creating a study plan is crucial when preparing for the CNA exam. Without one, you may feel overwhelmed and unsure of where to begin. The foremost step to passing the exam is creating a study plan is identifying how much time you have before your exam date.

Once you know this, create a schedule that maps out which topics or sections you must cover each day or week leading up to the exam. A plus point is giving yourself plenty of time for review and practice exams closer to the test date.

When creating your plan, consider what type of learner you are. Do you learn better by reading, listening, or doing? It will help determine the most effective materials and resources for studying.

It's also important to factor in breaks during your study sessions. Short breaks can improve productivity and retention when studying for long periods.

It's okay if things don't go according to plan sometimes - adjust as needed but stay committed! Creating a solid study plan now will pay off on exam day.

Gather study materials

Gathering study materials is one of the most essential steps in preparing for the CNA exam. But with so many resources available, choosing which ones to use can be overwhelming. Here are some tips on how to gather study materials effectively.

Firstly, start by reviewing the official test content outline provided by your state's nursing board, which will give you a roadmap of what topics you will cover in the exam. Once you've identified these areas, look for comprehensive textbooks or study guides that cover each case.

You can consult with online resources such as practice exams, and flashcards can also be beneficial when studying for the CNA exam. These tools allow candidates to review specific concepts repeatedly until they become familiar with them.

Remember other types of media, like videos or audio recordings, that can help make studying more engaging and interactive. Many online platforms offer free educational courses that cater specifically to CNA students.

Gathering too many materials may only sometimes be beneficial, too, since it might lead to information overload, which makes retention difficult. Focus only on high-quality materials relevant to your studies and avoid distractions from less valuable sources.

Ultimately, identifying quality study materials is a crucial step toward success in passing the CNA exam, and you must put effort into doing so before beginning your preparation efforts.

Study Strategy

When it comes to preparing for the CNA exam, having an effective study strategy is essential. Here are some guidelines to help you develop a successful study plan:

Firstly, identify your strengths and weaknesses. It will enable you to prioritize your studying accordingly.

Next, create a system of organization that works best for you. Whether it's flashcards or notes in a notebook, find what helps you retain information most effectively.

Another important aspect of your study strategy should be finding time to take practice tests. These tests can provide valuable insight into where you need more focus and familiarize you with the questions on the exam.

Additionally, consider forming a study group or utilizing online resources for support and additional learning opportunities.

Remember that everyone learns differently, with different abilities and IQ levels. You can experiment with other techniques until you find the best for your needs. With dedication and effort toward creating an effective study strategy, passing the CNA exam is achievable!

Create a study schedule

One of the primary things to do when preparing for the CNA exam is to create a study schedule. It will help you stay organized, ensure you get everything, and cover all the necessary topics before test day.

When creating your study schedule, identify how much time you have until your exam date. Then, decide how many hours you can study per day or week. Be realistic with yourself – remember that burning out won't help anyone.

Next, break down the topics into manageable sections and allocate time accordingly. For example, if there are six chapters in your textbook and four weeks until test day, aim to cover one chapter every three or four days.

Remember to build in breaks and rest days, too – giving yourself time off will improve your productivity in the long run.

Once you've created your study schedule, stick to it as best as possible. Of course, life happens sometimes, but having a clear plan can make it easier to get back on track after any disruptions.

Creating a study schedule may seem like an extra step, but it's worth its weight in gold when trying to prepare for an exam.

Utilize different study methods

When preparing for the CNA exam, utilizing different study methods is crucial. Everyone learns differently, so finding what works best for you is essential.

One method that may work well for visual learners is using flashcards or diagrams. These tools can help you memorize key concepts and terms through repetition and visualization.

For auditory learners, listening to lectures or recordings may be helpful. Many educational podcasts are available specifically for nursing students that cover various topics relevant to the CNA exam.

Another effective study method is group studying. It allows you to discuss and review material with peers with different perspectives and insights on the subject matter.

Practice exams are also valuable in test preparation as they simulate the actual testing environment and allow you to identify areas where further review is needed.

Incorporating different study methods into your routine can keep things interesting while helping you retain information more effectively. Remember, there's no one-size-fits-all approach – experiment with various techniques until you find the best compatible method.

Seek additional resources or support

Passing the CNA exam can be challenging, but with the proper preparation and study strategy, you can pass it with flying colors. Remember to create a plan that works for you, gather all necessary study materials, and schedule your time wisely.

Furthermore, don't hesitate to utilize different learning methods and seek additional resources or support when needed. It may include joining a study group or seeking tutoring services from experienced professionals.

Remember that passing the CNA exam is just one step towards achieving your career goals as a nursing assistant. When you do hard work and dedication, you can accomplish every challenge that comes your way in this rewarding profession. Best of luck on your journey!

Test-Taking Tips

Preparing for a test can be nerve-wracking, but you can breeze through the CNA exam with the correct strategies. Here are some steps to help you manage your time effectively and answer confidently.

First and foremost, make sure to read each question carefully before answering it. This way, you'll avoid making silly mistakes or misinterpreting what's asked. Additionally, if any information provides along with a question, such as graphs or tables, analyze them thoroughly.

Next up is managing your time wisely during the exam. You should spend proper time for each section based on its difficulty level, and don't get bogged down by difficult questions – move onto easier ones first, then come back later when you have more time.

While answering questions is important, it's equally essential not to guess answers mindlessly if uncertain since it could cost valuable marks. Instead of guessing randomly, eliminate options that seem unlikely until only one remains.

Review all your answers at least once before submitting the paper. It allows catching any errors or omissions made earlier in testing sessions while ensuring complete coverage of responses needed from candidates taking their exams under timed conditions.

Manage your time effectively

When it comes to taking the CNA exam, time management is crucial. You have limited time to answer all the questions, so you must use your minutes wisely.

One way to manage your time effectively is by setting your own pace. It is unnecessary to get bogged down on difficult questions and spend too much time on them. Instead, quickly move on and come back later if needed.

Another tip that can be effective time management during the CNA exam is to read each question carefully and thoroughly before answering. It can help prevent mistakes or misinterpretations that could waste valuable test-taking minutes.

Additionally, consider practicing with timed practice tests before the exam day arrives. It will show you how long it takes to answer specific questions and where you may need more focus during your study sessions.

Managing your time well during the CNA exam can create the difference between passing or failing. So, stay focused and keep a steady pace throughout!

Answer confidently but avoid guessing

When taking the CNA exam, it's essential to answer questions confidently. However, this doesn't mean that you should guess the answers. It's important to note that guessing can result in losing points if you get it wrong.

To avoid guessing, read each question carefully and try to understand what is being asked before answering. If you need more clarification about the answer, eliminate any incorrect choices, and then make an educated guess based on your knowledge of the subject matter.

If you're still uncertain after eliminating some choices, move on to another question and return later once you've answered other questions that may jog your memory or help provide context for what's asked.

Remember not to rush through questions because there is no penalty for leaving a question unanswered. Think critically and analyze each question thoroughly before providing an answer.

In addition, try not to second-guess yourself once you've selected an answer. Changing your initial response might lead to errors since, most likely initial responses are correct when made with enough thoughtfulness during reading comprehension.

By following these tips, answering confidently but avoiding guessing becomes more accessible, which increases the chances of passing the CNA exam!

Review your answers

Reviewing your answers is a crucial step in passing the CNA exam. Once you have completed all the questions, it's essential to take some time to check them over and make any necessary changes. Here are some tips on how to review your answers effectively:

Firstly, start by going through each question one at a time. Double-check that you have answered every question and that you have caught everything.

Next, read your answers carefully and look for any mistakes or inaccuracies. Check for spelling errors, incorrect grammar, or incomplete sentences.

It's also essential to ensure that you have understood each question correctly before answering it. Review the instructions provided with each question if necessary.

If you are still trying to find an answer but need help remembering specific details from your training materials, please double-check the information.

If there is still time left in the exam period after reviewing all of your answers thoroughly, consider reviewing some of the more challenging questions again and making any final adjustments as needed.

By taking these steps when reviewing your answers on the CNA exam, you can increase your chances of success while reducing stress levels during this critical moment.

Overcoming Test Anxiety

Test anxiety is a common problem that many people face when taking exams, including the CNA exam. It can cause feelings of fear and panic which can be overwhelming and prevent you from performing at your best. However, there are several techniques that you can use to overcome test anxiety.

Understand the causes of test anxiety:

The first step in overcoming test anxiety is to understand why it happens. Some possible causes include a lack of preparation, negative self-talk, fear of failure, or being judged by others.

Practice relaxation techniques:

Relaxation techniques such as deep breathing exercises, progressive muscle relaxation that calm yourself, and visualization exercises can help reduce symptoms of test anxiety. These practices promote calmness and mental clarity while relieving tension in your body.

Develop a positive mindset:

Positive thinking is critical to overcoming test anxiety. Instead of what could go wrong during the exam, focus on what you have already accomplished in your studies leading up to this point. Visualize yourself succeeding on the exam and remind yourself that you are capable.

Get adequate rest and self-care:

Sleeping before an exam is essential for promoting good physical health and mental alertness during testing. In addition to getting proper rest, engage in activities promoting self-care, such as exercise or listening to calming music.

By understanding the causes behind your test anxiety and utilizing these effective strategies for managing it, you will be better equipped to pass your CNA Exam confidently!

Understand the causes of test anxiety

Test anxiety is common for many students taking exams, including the CNA exam. It can transform into physical symptoms such as sweating and rapid heartbeat, leading to poor performance. To overcome test anxiety, it's essential to understand its causes.

One cause of test anxiety is fear of failure. Students may feel pressure from themselves or others to pass the exam, creating overwhelming stress and anxiety.

Another cause is a need for preparation. If a student feels unprepared or unsure about the material on the exam, they may become anxious when faced with difficult questions.

Additionally, past negative experiences with testing can contribute to test anxiety. If a student has failed previous exams or received poor grades in school, they may develop a fear and aversion towards taking tests.

To combat these causes of test anxiety, students should focus on building their confidence through adequate preparation and positive self-talk. Seeking support from friends or family can also help reduce stress levels before exams.

By understanding the root causes of test anxiety and implementing strategies to manage it effectively, CNA candidates have a better chance of passing their certification exam with flying colors!

Practice relaxation techniques

You can overcome test anxiety by practicing relaxation techniques. These techniques can help you relax your nerves and reduce stress levels.

One helpful technique is deep breathing exercises, which help slow down your heart rate and clear your mind. It would be an excellent idea to go to a quiet and calm place where you won't be disturbed, breathe profoundly and intensely through your nose for four seconds, and hold that breath for seven to nine seconds.

Then slowly exhale through your mouth for seconds. You can repeat this process several times until you feel more relaxed.

Another helpful technique is progressive muscle relaxation. It involves tensing and relaxing each muscle group, from the toes to the head. Focus on each area of tension as you tense it up for five to ten seconds before releasing it entirely while taking deep breaths.

Visualizations are also an excellent way to relax before an exam. Try picturing yourself in a peaceful environment, like sitting on a beach or walking in nature, while imagining all the sounds and sensations around you.

Make sure to practice these techniques regularly leading up to the exam day so that they become second nature when needed most!

Develop a positive mindset

A positive mindset is vital when preparing for the Certified Nursing Assistant (CNA) exam. A negative attitude can affect your confidence and performance, leading to poor results on the test. Here are some guidelines to help you cultivate a positive mindset.

Firstly, focus on your strengths rather than weaknesses. Recognize what you already know and have accomplished in your studies instead of worrying about what you don't know or haven't studied yet.

Secondly, avoid comparing yourself to others who may be taking the same exam as you. Everyone has unique strengths and challenges, so it's important not to measure yourself against someone else's progress.

Thirdly, visualize success by imagining yourself passing the CNA exam with flying colors. This mental practice can boost your confidence and motivate the actual test.

Surround yourself with positivity by seeking support from family members or friends who believe in you and encourage you. Their encouragement can further fuel your positive outlook toward success in passing this challenging exam.

In conclusion, passing the CNA exam requires diligent preparation, effective study strategies, and overcoming test anxiety. You can enhance your chances of success by following a structured study plan, understanding the exam requirements, and utilizing various study methods. Additionally, managing test anxiety through relaxation techniques, positive thinking, and self-care is crucial to perform at your best on exam day.

Remember to review the exam content thoroughly, allocate time wisely during the test, and answer questions confidently while avoiding guessing. Taking advantage of additional resources and seeking support from instructors and peers can also enhance your preparation.

Ultimately, consistent effort, self-belief, and a positive mindset will contribute to your success in the CNA exam. Stay focused, maintain discipline, and trust in your abilities. This exam will test your knowledge, and we wish you all the best in this career.

Chapter 3

Physical Care Skills

When you pass the exam and start your journey as a Certified Nursing Assistant (CNA), you play an essential role in providing physical care to patients. Your ability to assist patients with daily activities is vital for their health and well-being. When it comes to the CNA exam, mastering your physical care skills is crucial for passing the test and becoming a successful healthcare professional. This chapter will highlight the importance of physical care skills, explore what you can expect from the CNA exam regarding these skills, and provide helpful tips on how you can excel in personal care, dressing, grooming, nutrition, hydration, restoration of health, sleep and rest needs, elimination processes such as bowel movements or bladder control issues as well as addressing mobility concerns including destructive mobility issues among others. So, let's dive into this chapter on Physical Care Skills for CNA Exam!

The Importance of Physical Care Skills

Physical care skills are crucial for anyone working in the healthcare industry, especially for CNAs. These skills involve assisting patients with daily activities, such as bathing and dressing, feeding them, helping them use the bathroom, and moving around when necessary. CNAs help maintain their physical health by supporting patients while ensuring they receive quality care.

Moreover, physical care is essential in preventing complications from poor hygiene or lack of mobility. For instance, bedsores may develop if a patient is immobile for extended periods without being repositioned frequently enough. If left untreated or unnoticed by caregivers like CNAs who have training on these areas of concern during CNA exam preparation, bedsores can worsen quickly and lead to severe infections making it critical to understand how best to prevent such issues.

Caring for an individual's physical needs also significantly impacts their mental health and well-being. When patients feel clean and well-groomed, they tend to be more optimistic about themselves, which boosts their self-esteem and ultimately helps boost recovery rates after any medical intervention, including surgery and therapy sessions.

Mastering physical care skills as a CNA is not just about passing an exam but delivering quality holistic care that promotes physical and mental healing. It takes dedication and effort, but seeing your residents improve because you took exceptional care of them makes it all worth it.

The CNA Exam and Physical Care Skills

The Certified Nursing Assistant (CNA) exam is a crucial step for aspiring healthcare professionals who want to join the nursing field. The exam assesses candidates' knowledge and skills in various areas, including physical care skills. CNA aspirants must demonstrate their ability to perform tasks related to personal care, nutrition and hydration, mobility, elimination, circulation, and skin integrity.

To succeed in the CNA exam's physical care skills section, candidates must understand the importance of these skills. Physical care is integral to patient-centered care and involves meeting patients' basic needs while promoting health and well-being. Therefore, CNAs must possess excellent communication skills as they interact with patients daily.

CNAs should also be familiar with standard medical terminologies for accurately documenting patient records. It helps ensure continuity of care throughout the healthcare team.

Passing the CNA exam requires mastery of various physical care skill sets such as personal hygiene routines like bathing or grooming; proper mobilization techniques; preventing pressure sores through proper positioning or wound dressings; among others. Attention to detail and compassion go a long way when providing quality patient-centered services effectively and efficiently.

Personal care

Personal care is essential to a Certified Nursing Assistant's (CNA) job. It involves helping patients with daily self-care activities, such as bathing, grooming, and oral hygiene. CNAs must ensure patients feel comfortable during these personal activities and maintain their dignity.

Bathing is one of the most important aspects of personal care for patients who are immobile or bedridden. CNAs must assist them in sponge baths or showers, depending on the situation. During this process, it is crucial to have good communication skills to help make the patient feel more relaxed since they may be uncomfortable due to specific health conditions.

Grooming includes maintaining proper hair care by brushing and combing their hair regularly. For some patients who cannot perform these tasks themselves, CNAs can also provide shaving assistance for men and apply makeup for women when necessary.

CNAs should encourage independence in every activity while providing support whenever needed without undermining patient dignity or privacy.

Personal care is integral in ensuring a CNA provides optimal physical care services patients require under supervision throughout a healthcare facility.

Dressing and Grooming

Dressing and grooming are essential skills that CNAs must possess to care for their patients properly. These activities help maintain the patient's hygiene and promote a sense of dignity, self-respect, and independence.

When assisting with dressing, it is essential to ensure that the clothing is appropriate for the weather and fits comfortably. Respecting the patient's preferences concerning style, color, and dress material is crucial.

Grooming involves maintaining personal hygiene, such as bathing or showering regularly, brushing teeth twice daily, and combing the hair daily while keeping the patient's specific needs or preferences in mind. As a CNA, you must use safe practices when assisting with grooming tasks, such as using non-skid mats in wet areas like bathtubs.

CNAs should encourage patients to do as much as they can independently before assisting with dressing and grooming tasks. It helps promote independence among patients who otherwise may feel helpless without support.

In conclusion, mastering physical care skills such as dressing and grooming are vital competencies CNAs require during exam preparation. With these skills mastered correctly, comfort your clients while promoting self-esteem, ultimately improving overall mental health and well-being.

Nutrition and hydration

Nutrition and hydration are essential components of physical care skills that all CNAs need to master. Providing patients with adequate food and fluids is vital to maintaining their health, preventing dehydration, and facilitating healing.

A CNA must understand the patient's dietary restrictions and preferences to ensure proper nutrition. It involves knowing what foods to offer or avoid based on medical conditions such as diabetes or heart disease. It also includes paying attention to cultural norms, allergies, medication interactions, or religious practices that may impact a patient's food choices.

Hydration is equally important in maintaining good health. A CNA should encourage patients to drink enough water throughout the day while avoiding excessive caffeine or alcohol intake, as these can lead to dehydration.

In some cases, patients may require assistance with feeding due to physical limitations such as poor motor skills or cognitive deficits. CNAS must provide compassionate support while respecting the patient's dignity and independence.

Ensuring proper nutrition and hydration is critical in improving the well-being of those under our care as CNAs. By understanding each person's unique needs regarding diet and fluid intake, we can contribute significantly towards their recovery process while helping them maintain optimal health in both short-term hospitals stays through long-term assisted living arrangements.

Restoration and maintenance of health

Restoration and health maintenance are crucial physical care skills every CNA should have. As a nursing assistant, you must promote restoring and maintaining your patients' health through various means.

One way to achieve this goal is by helping the patient with their medication routine and ensuring they take their medications on time and as prescribed. You also need to monitor their vital signs regularly, which includes checking blood pressure, pulse rate, temperature, respiration rate, etc., for any changes or abnormalities.

Another essential aspect of restoring and maintaining health is assisting patients in performing exercises prescribed by physicians or therapists. These exercises help maintain muscle strength and mobility while promoting circulation throughout the body.

As a CNA, you will also provide emotional support to your patients. You can encourage them to participate in social activities such as games or reading books. It helps keep their minds sharp while giving them something fun to look forward to daily.

Maintaining cleanliness is crucial not only for personal hygiene but also for reducing hospital-acquired infections (HAIs). CNAs must ensure all surfaces are clean and disinfected since HAIs could cause further illness, delaying recovery times.

Sleep and rest needs

Sleep and rest are crucial components of physical care for healthcare patients, especially those receiving long-term care. As a CNA, you must understand the importance of quality sleep and rest to ensure your patient receives adequate rest.

Firstly, it is essential to note that each patient has unique sleep needs based on age, health status, medication use, and other factors. Therefore, as a CNA providing direct care to patients with varying conditions, it is essential to be observant and take feedback regarding their sleeping habits.

Promoting healthy sleeping patterns among patients under your care as a CNA requires creating an environment conducive to sleeping, such as dimming lighting or reducing noise levels. You can also encourage relaxation activities before bedtimes, such as light massage or reading books aloud.

If your patients experience difficulty falling or staying asleep despite practicing good sleep hygiene practices discussed above, communicate with RNs/LPNs about the possibility of administering medications prescribed by physicians authorized by law.

In summary, being aware of individualized sleep patterns and promoting good sleep hygiene practices will help avoid disruptions during bedtime routines while improving overall physical wellness among residents under your supervision.

Elimination (bowel and bladder)

Elimination is a fundamental aspect of human life, but it's also one of the most sensitive topics for patients and caregivers. As a CNA, you must master bowel and bladder elimination to provide quality patient care.

One crucial skill is recognizing signs of constipation or diarrhea. Patients with constipation may complain about abdominal pain, while those with diarrhea may experience frequent urges to use the toilet. CNAs should monitor bowel movements regularly and report any abnormalities or irregularities.

Another critical aspect is catheterization, which involves inserting a tube into the bladder through the urethra to remove urine. Catheters are often used on bedridden patients who can't get up frequently or have urinary incontinence issues.

CNAs must follow proper hygiene protocols when handling catheters, as improper insertion techniques could lead to infections and other complications. Mastering bowel and bladder elimination skills requires patience, attention to detail, and good communication skills with patients and healthcare professionals—essential traits for every successful CNA!

Mobility, including impaired mobility

Mobility is a crucial aspect of physical care skills for the CNA exam. It involves the ability to move around and perform daily activities with ease. However, mobility can be affected by various factors, such as injury, illness, or aging, resulting in lousy mobility.

Impaired mobility is characterized by difficulty moving around due to pain, stiffness, or weakness in muscles and joints. It can also lead to falls and other safety risks if not adequately addressed. As a CNA, you should be equipped with knowledge on how to assist patients with poor mobility.

To help patients improve their mobility, CNAs use different techniques such as range of motion exercises, gait training, and transfer techniques, among others. These techniques improve muscle strength, flexibility, and coordination while preventing further injuries.

In addition to these techniques, CNAS must provide and be familiar with assistive devices such as walkers or wheelchairs when necessary. It helps patients maintain independence while reducing the risk of falls or accidents.

Furthermore, providing emotional support is crucial when dealing with lousy mobility cases since it can affect a patient's self-esteem leading to depression or anxiety disorders.

Mastering the art of handling destructive mobility issues will make you an effective CNA capable of helping your patients achieve a better quality of life despite their health challenges.

Circulation and skin integrity

Circulation and skin integrity are critical physical care skills for CNAs to master. Proper circulation is essential for overall health, especially in older adults more prone to circulatory issues. As a CNA, monitoring the patient's blood pressure and pulse is necessary.

Skin integrity is another critical area of concern for CNAs. Individuals confined to their beds or with restricted movement may develop pressure ulcers called bedsores. These occur when there is prolonged pressure on bony areas such as the hips, tailbone, or heels. To prevent this from happening, CNAs should encourage patients to change positions frequently and assist with turning them over if necessary.

In addition to preventing bedsores, CNAs must watch for any signs of skin breakdown or irritation caused by incontinence products such as diapers or pads. Regularly changing these products and keeping the patient clean can help prevent infections and other complications.

Proper circulation and skin integrity are crucial components of physical care skills that all CNAs must learn to provide high-quality care for their patient's well-being.

Elimination (bladder and bowel)

As a certified nursing assistant (CNA), one of the most critical skills you must master is elimination care. It refers to assisting patients in maintaining healthy bowel and bladder function, essential for their overall well-being.

Regarding bowel elimination, CNAs should monitor their patients' regularity and consistency while promoting good hydration, fiber intake, and exercise. Constipation can lead to discomfort and even more severe problems, such as impaction or bowel obstruction.

Similarly, with bladder elimination, CNAs must ensure that their patients are adequately hydrated without overhydrating them. Adequate fluid intake helps prevent urinary tract infections (UTIs) and promotes healthy urine output volume and frequency.

It's also crucial for CNAs to maintain patient dignity when assisting with toileting needs. Patients may feel embarrassed or ashamed about needing help with these personal tasks, so always approach them with kindness, empathy, respect, and discretion.

Remember that every individual has unique toileting habits; some may require constant reminders while others need less prompting. Therefore it's crucial always to communicate effectively with your patient regarding their preferred bathroom routine.

Mastering physical care skills like elimination care requires patience and compassion toward your patient's individual needs - both physical & emotional needs to achieve the optimal health outcomes they deserve.

Patterns of Sleep and Rest

Caring for a patient's patterns of sleep and rest is an essential part of being a Certified Nursing Assistant (CNA). A patient's sleep quality can affect their overall physical and mental health. As CNAs, it is essential to understand the factors that may influence their patients' sleeping habits.

One crucial aspect to consider when caring for a patient's sleep pattern is their environment. Patients should be comfortable with a well-maintained bed, clean linens and blankets, and minimal noise or distractions.

Another factor impacting patients' rest time is pain management. Documenting any medication given is essential so other staff members know what has been administered is necessary.

The timing of meals can also play a role in sleep patterns; mealtimes should be consistent each day. Additionally, it's helpful to encourage some form of relaxation before bedtime, such as reading or listening to soothing music.

CNAs should communicate with patients regarding any issues related to their sleep cycle or schedule changes that have occurred recently. Understanding your patient's needs and preferences can help ensure they get the best night's rest possible under your care.

Self-image

Self-image is an essential aspect of physical care skills for CNA exams, affecting patients' mental and emotional well-being. It refers to how people perceive themselves based on appearance, abilities, and personality. As CNAs, part of our role is to help patients maintain a positive self-image.

We can do this by promoting personal hygiene. A clean and well-groomed appearance can boost patients' confidence and make them feel better about themselves. We should encourage patients to brush their teeth, comb their hair, and bathe regularly.

Another aspect of self-image that we need to consider is clothing. Patients should be able to wear clothes that fit comfortably and reflect their style. As CNAs, we can assist with dressing or provide adaptive clothing if necessary.

Additionally, communication plays a significant role in building a positive self-image for patients. We must listen when they express concerns or feelings about their health status or abilities without judgment.

As CNAs responsible for providing physical care skills for the CNA exam preparation process, we must promote healthy self-images in our patients through personal hygiene practices like grooming routines & assistance with adaptive clothing selection while also listening actively during interactions so they may feel valued as individuals beyond just what ailment(s) they face daily.

Strength and endurance

As a Certified Nursing Assistant (CNA), strength and endurance are crucial to providing quality patient care. The job requires physical strength, stamina, and the ability to lift heavy objects daily.

One way to build endurance and become physically stronger is by incorporating exercise into your daily routine. It can include walking or jogging, weight lifting, or stretching exercises. Building core strength through these types of activities will not only help you perform your job duties more efficiently but also prevent injury.

Maintaining a healthy diet is another essential factor in building physical strength and endurance. Eating protein-rich foods helps build muscle, while carbohydrates provide energy for physical activity. Staying hydrated with water throughout the day also supports optimal bodily function.

In addition to personal habits, following proper body mechanics when performing tasks like transferring patients from bed to chair or helping them walk around the room is essential. Correct techniques prevent strain on muscles and joints that could lead to injury over time.

Maintaining good health practices is critical to achieving optimal physical conditions as a CNA. By taking care of yourself first, you'll be able to better care for others who depend on you daily.

Care and use of assistive devices

As a CNA, you will be responsible and answerable for assisting patients with mobility and other activities of daily living. Sometimes, patients may require assistive devices to improve their overall function. You must understand how to properly care for and use these devices to ensure patient safety.

One standard assistive device is a wheelchair. When transferring or moving a patient in a wheelchair, always lock the wheels before attempting to communicate or stand them up. Also, ensure the footrests are securely in place so they don't accidentally fall off during transport.

Another type of assistive device is the walker. Walkers provide support and stability but must be used correctly to prevent falls or accidents. Encourage patients to keep their body weight centered over the walker for balance and always ensure it's adjusted at an appropriate height.

Canes are another popular device used by many people who need help, assistance, and care with balance or stability issues while standing or walking. Canes must have proper rubber tips on their base - worn-out tips can cause slips resulting in potential injuries.

In conclusion (oops!), knowing how to properly care for and use different assistive devices will help CNAs ensure patient safety and improve the overall quality of life.

Age-related changes

Age-related changes are a natural part of life that affects everyone differently. As people age, their bodies undergo several physiological changes that can impact their overall health and well-being. For example, many older adults experience decreased bone density, which increases the chances of fractures and falls.

Additionally, older individuals may have reduced muscle mass and strength, making it more challenging to perform daily tasks such as bathing or dressing independently. Hearing loss is also prevalent among seniors. It happens due to changes in the inner ear over time.

Cognitive changes are another aspect of aging that CNAs should be aware of. Memory decline is typical among older adults, especially regarding short-term memory recall. It can lead to confusion and forgetfulness for patients who are suffering from Alzheimer's disease or other forms of dementia.

Understanding these age-related changes is crucial for providing quality care to older adults as a CNA. Recognizing these challenges and adapting your approach while caring for them physically or emotionally will help ensure they receive the best care they deserve.

Cognitive changes

Cognitive changes are expected in aging adults and can affect their ability to perform daily tasks, communicate effectively, and maintain independence. These changes may range from mild forgetfulness to severe dementia.

One of the most significant cognitive changes is a decline in memory function. Older adults may experience difficulty recalling recent events or names of people they have recently met. They may also need help remembering important information, such as medication schedules or doctor's appointments.

In addition to memory problems, older adults may also experience a decline in problem-solving abilities and decision-making skills. It can make it challenging for them to plan or make choices independently.

Cognitive changes can also affect language processing, leading to difficulty communicating effectively with others. Some seniors might struggle to find the right words or express themselves clearly, which could lead to frustration and isolation.

It is essential for caregivers working with aging adults who have experienced cognitive changes to understand that these individuals need special attention and support when completing daily activities safely while maintaining some level of independence.

Psychosocial changes

Various psychosocial changes can affect our physical and emotional well-being as we age. Different factors, such as retirement, health issues, the death of loved ones, and social isolation, can cause these changes. As a CNA, understanding these changes is crucial in providing quality care to elderly patients.

One standard psychosocial change in older people is the feeling of loneliness brought about by social isolation. It can lead to depression and anxiety, which may require medication or therapy. CNAS need to provide companionship and establish a connection with their patients through active listening and engaging conversations.

Another significant psychosocial change associated with aging is the loss of independence due to physical limitations. This loss can impact an individual's self-worth, resulting in frustration or anger toward their current situation. As caregivers, it's essential to encourage participation in daily activities while respecting their personal choices.

Dementia-related conditions like Alzheimer's can cause significant psychosocial changes affecting patient behavior and mood swings leading to aggression outbursts against caregivers or other residents within communal living facilities.

In conclusion, awareness of these psychosocial challenges gives CNAs insight into how they should approach caregiving tasks effectively while fostering positive communication between themselves and older adults who need assistance maintaining dignity despite life-changing circumstances.

Physical changes

As we age, our bodies undergo various physical changes that can impact our daily lives and abilities. As a CNA, it is essential to understand these changes to provide the best possible care for your patients.

One significant physical change with aging is decreased muscle mass and strength. It can lead to difficulty with mobility and an increased risk of falls. As a CNA, you may need to assist your patients with walking or transferring from one place to another.

Another standard physical change is a decrease in vision and hearing. It can make it challenging for patients to communicate their needs or understand instructions given by healthcare providers. As a CNA, you may need to speak clearly and use visual aids such as written instructions or pictures.

Aging also often brings about changes in skin integrity, such as thinning skin and decreased elasticity. It increases the risk of pressure ulcers which require diligent monitoring by CNAs. You may need to reposition your patient frequently or ensure they use appropriate seat cushions.

In addition, many elderly individuals experience an increase in chronic conditions such as arthritis or cardiovascular disease which further impacts their physical abilities. It is essential for CNAs working with older adults to be aware of these conditions so they can provide appropriate care while minimizing discomfort.

Understanding these aging-related physical changes allows CNAs to adapt their care methods accordingly while providing compassionate support for their patients' individualized needs.

Psychosocial needs

As a CNA, it is essential to recognize the psychosocial needs of patients. These needs focus on emotional and social aspects of care that can significantly affect their well-being.

One key aspect of addressing psychosocial needs is establishing trust with patients. It involves active listening, empathy, and emotional support during difficult times. Patients who feel heard and understood are likelier to open up about their feelings and concerns.

Another important consideration when addressing psychosocial needs is respecting patients' cultural backgrounds. Understanding different customs and beliefs can help CNAs provide culturally competent care that meets each patient's needs.

Providing opportunities for socialization is also crucial in meeting psychosocial needs, especially for elderly or isolated patients. Encouraging group activities or arranging visits from family members can improve mood and overall quality of life.

Maintaining a positive attitude towards caregiving responsibilities will impact how you interact with your patient. A positive outlook will help create an environment where your patient feels safe and cared for.

Recognizing the importance of addressing psychosocial needs alongside physical care skills helps create a holistic approach to caregiving that promotes better health outcomes for patients.

It is a more demanding and challenging career. Your professional life as a Certified Nursing Assistant (CNA) requires more than just passing the exam. As a CNA, your foremost duty is to care for patients with age-related, cognitive, psychosocial, and physical changes requiring special attention.

As a CNA, it is your duty to provide quality patient care; it is essential to understand their unique needs and tailor your approach accordingly. It includes being knowledgeable about their physical care needs, such as hygiene and mobility assistance, and understanding their emotional needs by providing comfort and support.

By mastering these skills through education and hands-on experience, CNAs can make a significant difference in the lives of those they care for. Remember that being a CNA is about performing tasks and building meaningful relationships with patients.

So if you are considering pursuing this career path or preparing for the CNA exam, remember to focus on developing your technical and interpersonal skills. With dedication and commitment to delivering exceptional patient care, you can become an invaluable member of any healthcare team.

Chapter 4

Nursing Care

Nursing care is a delicate point of a CNA's professional life. This work contains many technicalities. So, understanding the importance of observation and reporting in nursing care is crucial! As a certified nursing assistant (CNA), your role involves:

- Closely monitoring patients' physical changes.
- Documenting them accurately.
- Reporting any concerns to other healthcare professionals.

This chapter dives deeper into the significance of observation and reporting in nursing care. We'll also explore essential techniques for observing physical changes, report methods and documentation, case studies, practice scenarios related to major body systems, and joint disorders related to each design. So, let's get started!

Duties of a CNA

As a CNA, your primary duty is to provide essential care and support to patients who cannot perform their daily activities. As such, you will often have the most significant amount of interaction with patients in a healthcare setting. You'll be responsible for ensuring that they receive appropriate care, comfort, and safety.

One of the core duties of CNAs is assisting patients with daily activities like bathing and dressing. This task requires an understanding of both hygiene practices and personal preferences.

In addition to essential patient care duties, CNAs must regularly monitor vital signs such as blood pressure, heart rate, temperature levels, etc. They must report any changes in these parameters to medical staff promptly.

Another crucial responsibility is maintaining accurate records regarding each patient's condition or progress during treatment. These updates help physicians track how well treatment plans are working so that adjustments can be made if necessary.

CNAs should also keep detailed notes on everything from medications administered to food intake & output (to ensure proper hydration). Doing this helps prevent potential complications later on in treatment.

Being a CNA comes with many responsibilities - from helping older adults get dressed daily to monitoring vital signs frequently; it takes hard work but ultimately rewarding knowing that you're positively impacting someone's life!

Importance of observation and reporting in nursing care

As a CNA, compliance, and reporting are essential to your role. The ability to closely monitor and accurately document patients' physical changes is crucial for ensuring they receive the best care. Observing patients involves using your senses, such as sight, touch, hearing, and smell, to check their condition continually.

One of the most critical reasons observation is vital in nursing care is detecting any changes that may indicate a decline in health status. Early detection can help prevent complications or save lives by enabling timely interventions before conditions worsen.

Another reason why observing patients is essential in CNA practice is that it helps identify patterns that could point toward specific disorders or illnesses. Documenting these observations records the patient's history, which can be used for future reference when making diagnoses or providing treatment options.

Reporting observations accurately also plays an integral part in nursing care since healthcare professionals rely on this information to make informed decisions about the treatments required. Accurate documentation enables other healthcare professionals to provide high-quality care based on precise patient needs information.

Observation and reporting are fundamental aspects of nursing care that should always be noticed by CNAs or anyone involved in providing quality healthcare services. Through close monitoring and proper documentation practices, we can offer better patient outcomes while improving overall health service delivery standards.

Observation and Reporting Physical Changes

As a Certified Nursing Assistant (CNA), one of your primary duties is to observe and report any physical changes in a patient's health. It involves being attentive to the patient's body temperature, skin color, vital signs, mobility issues, and overall appearance. The details are mentioned below.

Definition and importance of physical changes

When it comes to nursing care, physical changes are an essential aspect that must be monitored and reported. Material changes refer to any alterations in the body's appearance or function. These can range from simple cuts and bruises to more complex issues like chronic illnesses.

The importance of physical changes lies in their ability to provide valuable insights into a patient's health status. By observing these changes, nurses can detect potential problems early on and take necessary actions before they escalate into severe conditions.

To effectively observe physical changes, there are several techniques that nurses can use. It includes regular assessments of vital signs such as blood pressure, pulse rate, and temperature. Other methods involve monitoring skin color, texture, and moisture level.

Reporting methods for physical changes also play a critical role in nursing care. Nurses must accurately document all observations made during their shifts using clear language and appropriate medical terminology. It ensures that other healthcare professionals who may attend to the patient have access to complete information about their condition.

Understanding the definition of physical changes is crucial for any nurse providing quality care. Identifying these changes through accurate observation techniques is critical in preventing complications or identifying potential issues early on. At the same time, proper documentation helps ensure continuity of care throughout different shifts by various healthcare providers involved with the patient's treatment plan.

Techniques for observing physical changes

As a nursing assistant, observing physical changes in patients is an essential part of your job. These observations can help identify potential health concerns and ensure prompt intervention. Here are some techniques to help you make accurate observations:

Firstly, use your senses to gather information about the patient's appearance, behavior, and environment. It includes noticing changes in their skin color or texture, breathing patterns, body temperature, and movement.

Secondly, please communicate with the patient to gather more detailed information about their symptoms or discomforts. Ask open-ended questions such as "How are you feeling today?" or "Do you have any pain?"

Thirdly, monitor vital signs regularly using appropriate equipment like blood pressure cuffs and thermometers. Record these measurements accurately for reference by other healthcare professionals.

Be vigilant when performing routine tasks like bathing or feeding patients. You should keep a check on the patient's history and observe for any new bruises or injuries saw them.

Being attentive and thorough when observing physical changes is crucial for providing quality care to patients.

Reporting methods and documentation

Reporting methods and documentation are essential aspects of nursing care. It involves recording all the patient's health record observations to ensure that everyone involved in their treatment is aware of any changes or trends. Adequate documentation also ensures continuity of care between shifts and promotes more effective communication among healthcare providers.

Nurses should be accurate, concise, objective, and timely when documenting patients' information. It includes ensuring that they write legibly and use appropriate medical terminology. Documentation should also indicate the observer's date, time, location, name, and any interventions performed.

Different reporting methods are available for nurses depending on the situation at hand. These include SBAR (Situation-Background-Assessment-Recommendation), PIE (Problem-Intervention-Evaluation), and SOAP (Subjective-Objective-Assessment-Plan), among others.

Additionally, it is crucial to protect patient privacy during documentation by adhering to HIPAA regulations while accessing electronic health records or communicating with other healthcare team members about a patient's condition.

Proper reporting methods and thorough documentation are critical to providing quality nursing care. Accurate records help improve patient outcomes by facilitating efficient communication between healthcare providers leading to comprehensive, holistic care plans for each aspect of a patient's needs.

Case studies and practice scenarios

As a nursing assistant, it's essential to be prepared for any situation. That's why case studies and practice scenarios are crucial in helping CNAs develop their skills and knowledge.

Case studies provide real-life examples of patient care situations where you can learn how to handle certain conditions or symptoms. These scenarios test your ability to think critically, prioritize tasks, and communicate effectively with patients, family members, and other healthcare professionals.

Practice scenarios allow you to apply the theoretical knowledge you have learned in a controlled environment. You can practice taking vital signs accurately or responding appropriately during an emergency.

Regularly participating in these exercises will make you more confident in handling various patient care situations. You'll also learn from your mistakes so that you know what actions to take when faced with similar circumstances again.

It's essential not only to memorize procedures but also to understand the reasoning behind them. Case studies and practice scenarios provide practical experience that can help bridge this gap between theory and reality.

Basic Anatomy and Functions of Body Systems

As a certified nursing assistant (CNA), it is essential to know the basic anatomy and functions of the human body. It helps in understanding how different systems work together to maintain overall health.

Overview of major body systems

The human body is a complex machine of several systems that work together to keep us alive and healthy. Understanding these systems is essential for any nurse or nursing assistant. This section will guide CNAs about effective body systems.

Firstly, the respiratory system. It is about the lungs and airways and helps us breathe in oxygen and expel carbon dioxide. Next is the circulatory system, which pumps blood through the heart, arteries, veins, and capillaries.

The digestive system processes food into nutrients that our bodies can absorb. It consists of organs such as the mouth, esophagus, stomach, intestines, liver, and pancreas.

The nervous system controls all bodily functions using electrical impulses sent through neurons in our brains and spinal cord. The endocrine system produces hormones to regulate physiological functions like growth or metabolism.

Muscular-skeletal System gives structure to our body and enables movement through muscles attached to bones via tendons. At the same time, the skin acts as a protective barrier against bacteria or injury while regulating temperature through sweat glands.

Last but not least immune, lymphatic system plays a crucial role in fighting infections by identifying foreign substances entering our bodies.

Understanding each body's function provides insight into how they interconnect with one another, promoting overall health for individuals across their lifespans.

Anatomy and functions of each body system

The human body is an intricate and complex system comprising various organs, tissues, and cells that work together to keep us alive. Each body system has a unique anatomy and function, contributing to an individual's health and well-being.

The circulatory is about the heart, blood vessels, and blood. Its primary function is transporting oxygenated blood from the lungs to all body parts while removing carbon dioxide waste products.

The respiratory system includes the lungs, trachea, bronchi, alveoli, and diaphragm. It's responsible for exchanging gases between our bodies and the environment by inhaling oxygen-rich air into our lungs while exhaling carbon dioxide waste.

The digestive system comprises several organs, such as the stomach, intestines, liver, pancreas gallbladder, which work together to break down food into small nutrient molecules so your body can absorb them.

Another important system is the musculoskeletal, which comprises bones, muscles, joints, tendons, ligaments cartilage. It provides structural support for movement providing flexibility, strength, stability, balance, coordination, posture, and protecting inner organs.

All these systems have vital roles in keeping us physically and mentally healthy; each has functions that contribute to optimal well-being. Understanding how they work can help individuals make informed decisions about their healthcare choices.

Characteristics of Body Functions

As a CNA, you'll monitor various body functions to ensure your patients are healthy and comfortable. Understanding the characteristics of normal and abnormal body functions is crucial in identifying any changes that may indicate illness or injury.

Normal body functions include a range of vital signs such as temperature, blood pressure, pulse rate, and respiration rate. These values can differ depending on age, physical activity level, and other factors.

Abnormal body functions can present themselves in different ways. For example, an elevated temperature could indicate infection, while low blood pressure could indicate dehydration or shock.

Assessing and monitoring these vital signs will be essential for quality patient care. By recognizing subtle changes early on through regular observation and promptly reporting any concerns to the nursing team, you can help prevent further complications.

Normal body functions and vital signs

As a nursing assistant, it's essential to understand patients' normal body functions and vital signs.

Vital signs are important indicators of overall health status and can help detect early warning signs of illness or disease. The four primary vital signs include body temperature, blood pressure, pulse rate, and respiratory rate.

Average body temperature ranges from 97°F to 99°F (36.1°C to 37.2°C) in adults but may vary depending on age and other factors. Blood pressure readings typically range between 90/60 mm Hg to 120/80 mm Hg for most adults at rest.

Pulse rate refers to the heart beats per minute and can be felt at various points throughout the body, such as the wrist or neck. A healthy adult usually has a resting heart rate between 60-100 beats per minute.

The respiratory rate measures how many breaths a person takes in one minute while at rest. Standard adult rates are typically between 12-20 breaths per minute but vary based on age and activity level.

By understanding what is considered "normal" for each vital sign measurement, CNAs can recognize when there is an abnormality that should be reported promptly to their nursing team. Accurate documentation of these measurements is crucial for providing quality care that meets patients' needs effectively.

Abnormal body functions and signs of illness

The nursing team should always be on the lookout for abnormal body functions and signs of illness. These signs can vary depending on the patient's age, medical history, and current condition.

Some standard abnormal body functions include changes in heart rate, blood pressure, temperature, breathing patterns, and pain levels. For example, a rapid heart rate may indicate an infection or dehydration, while high blood pressure may point to cardiovascular disease.

Other signs of illness may manifest as physical symptoms such as rashes, swelling, disorientation, or Confusion. Patients with chronic conditions like diabetes may also experience fluctuations in their glucose levels which could cause several symptoms, including dizziness or fatigue.

As a CNA caregiver, it is essential to take note of these early indications of health problems so that appropriate interventions can make promptly. It will help prevent complications from arising while ensuring optimal recovery for patients.

Assessing and monitoring body functions

Assessing and monitoring body functions is a crucial aspect of nursing care. The CNAs need to understand the normal range of signs like blood pressure, pulse rate, respiratory rate, temperature, and oxygen saturation to identify any sudden abnormalities that may indicate an underlying health issue.

Nurses should gather information about the patient's medical history and current medications during assessments. They must also observe skin color and condition, listen for lung or gut sounds with a stethoscope, check pupils' reactions to light changes, and assess mobility or balance issues.

In addition to these assessments, nurses regularly monitor patients throughout their shifts by checking vital signs. If there are any significant changes outside of the norm or if symptoms worsen despite treatment interventions over time, they must notify the physician immediately.

Nurses also need to document all observations accurately using precise language. This documentation helps other healthcare professionals make informed decisions regarding patient care while ensuring continuity between shifts.

Assessing and monitoring body functions is essential in identifying early warning signs of illness, allowing prompt intervention when needed, ultimately leading to improved patient outcomes.

Recognizing and reporting changes in body functions

Recognizing and reporting changes in body functions is a crucial aspect of nursing care. Being a Certified Nursing Assistant (CNA), you must identify signs indicating that the patient's body function has changed. These could include changes in temperature, pulse rate, respiratory rate, or blood pressure.

One way to recognize these changes is by regularly monitoring the patient's vital signs and comparing them with previous recordings. It can help detect any deviation from normal levels early on. Attention to other physical symptoms, such as pain, nausea, or difficulty breathing, is also essential.

Once you have identified any changes in the patient's body functions, it is essential to report them promptly to the nursing team. Accurate documentation of these observations will ensure that appropriate interventions implement quickly.

As a CNA, your alertness and timely reporting can significantly prevent further patient complications. Therefore, always watch for changes in their body functions and communicate effectively with other healthcare professionals involved in their care plan.

Observation and Reporting of Behavior Changes

Observation and reporting of behavior changes are crucial aspects of nursing care. Nurses must pay close attention to their patients' behaviors, as changes in behavior can indicate underlying medical issues or emotional distress.

Understanding behavior changes in patients requires careful observation and documentation. Techniques for observing include watching the patient's facial expressions, body language, and verbal responses. It is essential to document any observed behavior changes accurately using precise descriptions.

Communication strategies with patients exhibiting behavioral changes are also critical. Nurses should approach these interactions with empathy and understanding while maintaining professional boundaries. The nurse should provide a safe environment that encourages open communication by actively listening to the patient.

Reporting any observed behavioral changes to the nursing team is vital for effective care coordination. Early behavior change detection can prevent further complications, improving patient outcomes.

In summary, nurses are essential in observing and documenting behavioral changes and communicating effectively with patients experiencing such challenges. Reporting these observations ensures that healthcare providers take necessary measures to provide optimal care for their patients' improved health outcomes.

Understanding behavior changes in patients

Understanding patient behavior changes is crucial to providing high-quality nursing care. Patients may exhibit various behaviors indicating their current emotional or mental state, including agitation, Confusion, sadness, or aggression.

As nurses, it's essential to understand the underlying causes behind these behaviors. For example, patients with dementia may become agitated due to feelings of fear or disorientation. Similarly, individuals experiencing chronic pain might display irritability and frustration.

Observing and documenting these behavioral changes is also essential for effective communication between healthcare professionals. Nurses must have clear documentation of any observed changes in behavior so that other medical team members can make informed decisions about patient care.

Developing robust communication strategies with patients experiencing behavioral changes is equally important as understanding them. Active listening and empathy are critical tools for building patient trust and helping them feel heard during difficult times.

In summary, understanding patient behavior changes requires careful observation skills combined with empathy and effective communication techniques. By utilizing all three components as part of an overall nursing strategy, healthcare providers can improve patient outcomes while promoting greater well-being across the medical community.

Techniques for observing and documenting behavior changes

Observing and documenting behavior changes is essential to a nursing assistant's job. It helps identify potential issues or problems that may arise with the patient. Here are some techniques for observing and documenting behavior changes.

Firstly, it's essential to establish baseline behaviors for each patient. It means taking note of their usual demeanor, communication style, and daily routine. By selecting a baseline, we can more easily identify when something unexpected occurs.

Secondly, observation should do non-intrusively not to disrupt the patient's everyday activities or behaviors. As nursing assistants, we need to be vigilant without being overly invasive.

Thirdly, it is crucial to document behavioral changes accurately and thoroughly, including what was observed and when it occurred. The documentation must also include information about any interventions taken by staff members.

Good communication skills are vital when reporting observations to other healthcare team members; clear descriptions will help others understand what has been noted during your comments.

Observing and documenting behavior changes requires skillful techniques while respecting the patient's privacy and dignity. These methods ensure accurate identification of potential risks or issues while providing valuable insight into our patients' well-being over time.

Changes in Mental Status (Confusion)

Being a certified nursing assistant (CNA), it is vital to identify changes in mental status, particularly Confusion. Confusion causes a variety of factors, such as medication side effects or underlying medical conditions.

Definition and causes of mental status changes

Mental status changes alter a person's cognitive, emotional, and behavioral functioning. These changes may be unexpected or gradual and can manifest as Confusion, disorientation, agitation, aggression, anxiety, or depression. The causes of mental status changes can vary widely depending on the patient's health history.

Physical conditions such as infections, nutritional deficiencies, or traumatic brain injury can cause mental status changes. Medications prescribed for various medical conditions, like painkillers and sedatives, may also affect a person's mental state.

In elderly patients with dementia or Alzheimer's, cognitive decline may lead to Confusion and disorientation. Patients undergoing treatment for cancer experience fatigue which can impact their concentration levels leading to mental status changes.

Nurses must understand the potential causes of mental status changes to provide appropriate care that addresses the underlying issue rather than just treating symptoms alone. By identifying the root cause of these issues, CNAs can develop an effective treatment plan to work on the patient's overall health while reducing adverse side effects associated with different treatments available today.

Signs and symptoms of Confusion

When it comes to nursing care, identifying signs and symptoms of Confusion is essential. Various factors, including medication side effects, infections, or medical conditions like dementia, can cause the disorder.

Some common signs and symptoms of Confusion include disorientation to time or place, difficulty following conversations or instructions, memory loss, and changes in behavior. Patients may also exhibit physical signs such as restlessness or agitation.

Nurses need to assess patients regularly for Confusion and note any changes in mental status. It helps ensure early intervention if necessary.

If a patient is confused, the nurse must take steps to create a calm environment and provide reassurance. Speaking slowly and clearly while using simple language can help reduce anxiety levels.

Recognizing Confusion signs allows nurses to understand their patients' needs better and provide appropriate care.

Techniques for assessing and monitoring mental status

Evaluating and monitoring mental status is an essential part of nursing care. The CNAs ensure that patients receive appropriate care; it's vital to identify the potential causes for Confusion or altered mental status. The CNAs should be able to recognize signs and symptoms of cognitive impairment as early as possible.

One way to assess a patient's mental status is through standardized tools such as the Mini-Mental Status Examination (MMSE) or Montreal Cognitive Assessment (MoCA). These tools evaluate various aspects of cognition, including orientation, memory, language, attention, and more.

Observation also plays a crucial role in assessing mental status changes. It includes observing behavior patterns like speech patterns, motor skills, and mood changes. Additionally, asking open-ended questions can help elicit helpful information about how a patient is feeling.

The CNAs need to monitor their patient's mental state throughout their stay at the healthcare facility continuously. Regular screening helps detect any new developments in cognitive function promptly.

Utilizing subjective observation techniques and standard assessments can provide valuable insights into a patient's overall condition while ensuring high-quality nursing care.

Orientation/Validation Techniques

Being a certified nursing assistant is both challenging and rewarding. Providing care to patients requires dedication, compassion, and attention to detail. A CNA's responsibilities are critical in ensuring patients receive the best care.

Importance of orientation and validation in patient care

As a nursing assistant, providing comprehensive care to patients is essential. One crucial aspect of patient care is the importance of direction and validation. Exposure refers to helping patients understand their surroundings, while validation affirms patients' feelings and emotions.

Patients feeling lost or confused in an unfamiliar environment may experience anxiety and fear. That's why it's crucial for nursing assistants always to orient them by explaining where they are, what they can expect during their stay, and who will be taking care of them.

Validation is also critical, as many patients may feel overwhelmed with their condition or situation. Nursing assistants should empathize with their feelings while providing reassurance that they are not alone.

Nursing assistants can foster trust and build patient relationships by practicing orientation and validation techniques daily. This approach creates a supportive atmosphere which helps put the patient at ease during treatment- ultimately enhancing overall patient satisfaction levels.

Orientation & Validation techniques go beyond just caring for physical needs; it involves creating emotional support for individuals experiencing life changes due to illness or injury- all contributing significantly towards achieving holistic healing outcomes.

Techniques for orienting and validating patients

As a nursing care provider, orienting and validating patients is essential to your job. It helps to establish trust and create a sense of security for the patient.

One technique for orientation is providing visual cues such as calendars, clocks, or signs that display the date, time, and location. It helps reduce Confusion in patients with difficulty remembering important details.

Another method is verbal reassurance which involves speaking calmly and clearly while maintaining eye contact with the patient. Repeat instructions if necessary and encourage them to ask questions whenever they feel unsure about something.

Validation techniques involve acknowledging your patient's feelings by offering empathy or showing concern when they express their emotions. It can do through active listening, where you give undivided attention to what they are saying without interrupting or rushing them.

It's essential also to use positive reinforcement by praising them for any efforts made towards their recovery, regardless of how small it may seem. By doing this, you boost their self-esteem, which directly impacts their overall well-being.

Orienting and validating patients requires patience, empathy, clear communication skills, and creativity in finding effective ways that work best for each patient's needs.

Strategies for providing a supportive environment

A supportive environment is crucial when caring for patients experiencing mental status changes. It can help them feel safe and secure, which in turn can aid their recovery process. Here are some plans that you can use to create a supportive environment:

Firstly, it's essential to maintain a calm and peaceful atmosphere in the patient's room or ward. You can achieve this by decreasing noise levels, using soft lighting, and playing relaxing music.

Secondly, establish rapport with your patient by conversing with them and showing genuine interest in their well-being. It will help build trust between you and the patient.

Another strategy is encouraging family members or loved ones to visit the patient regularly. Having visitors can provide emotional support for the patient and improve their mood.

Ensure patients can access activities they enjoy, such as reading books or watching movies. These activities can distract them from negative thoughts and improve their overall well-being.

By implementing these strategies, you'll provide an environment where patients feel comfortable sharing their feelings while aiding in faster recovery times.

Case studies and role-playing exercises

Case studies and role-playing exercises are valuable for CNAs to develop critical thinking skills. By presenting real-life scenarios, case studies allow students to apply the knowledge learned in class and identify potential solutions. Role-playing exercises help students practice patient communication and learn how to handle difficult situations.

In a nursing care context, case studies can cover various topics, such as medication administration errors, falls prevention strategies, or patient-centered care planning. Students may be asked to analyze the situation from different angles, discuss possible interventions with their peers or write up a care plan based on their findings.

Role-playing exercises often involve acting out common scenarios that CNAs encounter in hospital settings, such as communicating with non-English speaking patients or dealing with angry family members. These activities enable students to gain confidence in their communication skills and test new approaches before applying them in real-world situations.

Both case studies and role-playing exercises offer an interactive way for nursing students to learn about best practices while developing critical problem-solving skills needed for success as healthcare professionals.

Emotional Stress

As a CNA, you'll encounter patients who are going through different types of emotional stress. These can range from anxiety and depression to fear and anger. It's essential to understand that emotional stress affects people differently, so empathy toward their situation is crucial.

Understanding emotional stress and its impact on patients

Emotional stress can significantly impact a patient's overall health and well-being. Emotional stress can cause physical symptoms such as headaches, muscle tension, and fatigue, whether due to illness, injury, or other life events. It can also affect the immune system and increase the risk of developing chronic diseases.

As healthcare providers, we must recognize the signs of emotional stress in our patients. Some common indicators include changes in mood or behavior, difficulty sleeping or concentrating, feelings of anxiety or hopelessness, and increased use of drugs or alcohol.

Providing support and coping strategies is crucial when caring for patients experiencing emotional stress. It may involve encouraging relaxation techniques such as deep breathing exercises or recommending counseling services for those who need additional assistance.

It's also essential to create an environment that promotes healing by reducing sources of stress wherever possible—adjusting visitation policies to allow more time with loved ones or minimizing noise levels within hospitals and clinics.

By understanding the impact of emotional stress on our patients' health outcomes and taking steps to provide appropriate care and support, we can help them achieve optimal recovery while improving their quality of life overall.

Mood Status Changes

A. Definition and Causes of Mood Status Changes:

1. **Definition:** Mood status changes refer to fluctuations or alterations in a person's emotional state, including shifts in mood, affect, and overall emotional well-being. These changes can manifest as energy levels, motivation, interest, and overall vibrant tone variations.

2. **Causes of Mood Status Changes:** a. Biological Factors: Biological factors play a significant role in mood regulation. Hormonal imbalances, such as during hormonal

cycles or menopause, can influence mood stability. Fluctuations in neurotransmitters, such as serotonin and dopamine, can also impact mood. Additionally, genetic predispositions may make specific individuals more susceptible to mood fluctuations and mood disorders.

3. **Psychological Factors:** Psychological factors can profoundly impact mood status. Stress-related to work, personal relationships, or financial concerns can lead to mood disturbances. Traumatic experiences, such as accidents or the loss of a loved one, can trigger mood changes, including symptoms of depression or anxiety. Furthermore, individuals with preexisting mental health conditions, such as depression or bipolar disorder, may experience more pronounced and frequent mood status changes.

4. **Environmental Factors:** Environmental factors can contribute to mood fluctuations. Lack of social support, isolation, or unhealthy relationships can negatively affect mood and emotional well-being. Exposure to chronic stressors, such as ongoing work-related pressures or living in an unsafe environment, can also impact mood. Lifestyle factors, including poor nutrition, inadequate sleep, and limited physical activity, can influence mood stability.

B. Assessing and Monitoring Mood Status:

Assessing and monitoring mood status is crucial for identifying mood changes and providing appropriate care. Here are some methods for assessing and monitoring mood status:

1. **Patient Interview:** Engage in open and empathetic communication with the patient to understand their current emotional state. Ask about their feelings, emotions, and any recent changes in mood or behavior. Please encourage them to express themselves openly, providing a safe and non-judgmental environment for disclosure.

2. **Observation:** Observe the patient's non-verbal cues, like facial expressions, body language, and tone of voice. Look for sadness, irritability, agitation, or other emotional indicators. Pay attention to changes in energy levels, sleep patterns, appetite, and social interactions.

3. **Mood Assessment Tools:** Utilize standardized mood assessment tools like questionnaires or scales to gather more objective information. Examples include the Beck Depression Inventory (BDI), the (HAM-D), and the Geriatric Depression Scale (GDS). These tools provide a systematic way to assess and monitor mood changes over time.

4. **Collaborative Approach:** Involve the patient's support system, including family members, caregivers, and healthcare professionals, in the assessment and monitoring process. They may provide valuable insights into the patient's mood status, mainly if they have observed changes over an extended period.

C. Techniques for Promoting Positive Mood and Emotional Well-being:

Nurses and healthcare providers play a vital role in promoting positive mood and emotional well-being. Here are some techniques to enhance a patient's perspective:

1. **Active Listening and Emotional Support:** Practice listening to understand and validate the patient's emotions. Provide a supportive and non-judgmental environment where patients feel comfortable expressing their feelings. Show empathy and offer reassurance to reduce emotional distress.

2. **Therapeutic Communication:** Use effective communication techniques to establish a therapeutic relationship with the patient. Encourage open dialogue, ask open-ended questions, and provide opportunities for patients to discuss their concerns. Validate their experiences and provide real hope and encouragement.

Defense Mechanisms

A. Overview of Defense Mechanisms in Psychology:

1. **Defense Mechanisms:** Defense mechanisms are essential in psychological strategies that individuals employ unconsciously to protect themselves from anxiety, emotional distress, and threatening thoughts or situations. They serve as coping mechanisms that help individuals maintain psychological equilibrium and preserve self-esteem.

2. **Freudian Theory:** A prominent psychologist, Sigmund Freud, introduced the concept of defense mechanisms called psychoanalytic theory. According to Freud, defense mechanisms operate unconsciously and involve various psychological processes that modify, distort, or deny reality to alleviate anxiety.

B. Recognizing and Understanding Common Defense Mechanisms:

1. **Repression:** Repression involves the unconscious exclusion of distressing thoughts, memories, or feelings from conscious awareness. Individuals may repress traumatic experiences or unacceptable desires to avoid emotional pain.

2. Denial means to accept or acknowledge reality or truth that may be psychologically distressing. Individuals in denial may dismiss evidence or rationalize situations to maintain their preferred validity.

3. Projection occurs when individuals attribute their unacceptable thoughts, feelings, or motives to others. By projecting these traits onto others, individuals can avoid acknowledging and dealing with them in themselves.

4. Rationalization involves creating logical or plausible explanations to justify or excuse one's behavior, actions, or feelings. It allows individuals to maintain self-esteem and reduce guilt or anxiety associated with their choices.

5. **Displacement:** Displacement involves redirecting one's emotions or impulses from their source to a substitute target that is less threatening or more accessible. For example, someone angry with their boss may focus their frustration on their family members instead.

6. **Sublimation:** Sublimation channels or transforms socially unacceptable impulses or behaviors into more socially acceptable forms. For instance, an individual with aggressive tendencies may find release and expression through sports or creative pursuits.

7. **Regression:** Regression involves reverting to earlier stages of development or behaving in childlike ways when facing stressful or challenging situations. This defense mechanism temporarily relieves anxiety but can hinder personal growth and problem-solving.

8. Intellectualization entails approaching a situation or emotion detached and analytically, emphasizing facts and logic while suppressing the associated feelings. It allows individuals to distance themselves from the emotional impact of the crisis.

C. Interactions between Defense Mechanisms and Patient Care:

1. **Awareness and Recognition:** Healthcare providers should know defense mechanisms and recognize when patients may employ them. Understanding defense mechanisms can help caregivers interpret patients' behaviors, emotions, and responses more accurately, leading to more effective care.

2. **Communication and Therapeutic Relationship:** Recognizing defense mechanisms can inform the approach and style of communication with patients. By creating a non-judgmental and supportive environment, healthcare providers can encourage patients to explore their defenses, challenge maladaptive ones, and develop healthier coping strategies.

3. **Emotional Support:** Patients may employ defense mechanisms to manage overwhelming emotions and protect themselves. Healthcare providers should offer empathy, validation, and emotional support to help patients feel safe and understood. It can foster trust and facilitate patients' willingness to explore their emotions more openly.

4. **Treatment Planning:** Understanding the defense mechanisms patients utilize can inform the development of individualized treatment plans. By addressing the symptoms and underlying psychological defenses, healthcare providers can support patients in achieving meaningful and lasting change.

Acute emergencies

Acute emergencies are a common occurrence in the healthcare industry. It requires quick thinking and immediate action to ensure optimal patient outcomes. Being calm and collected during these situations is essential as a CNA professional while assessing and prioritizing the patient's needs.

One example of an acute emergency is cardiac arrest. In this case, every second counts as the heart has stopped beating, depriving vital organs of oxygen-rich blood. Nurses must initiate cardiopulmonary resuscitation (CPR) immediately to restore blood flow and prevent brain damage.

Another example is anaphylaxis or severe allergic reactions where patients may experience difficulty breathing, swelling of their face or throat, hives or rash on their skin with itching sensation, among other symptoms. Administering epinephrine through intramuscular injection can quickly resolve these symptoms.

Moreover, stroke patients require immediate evaluation for appropriate interventions such as clot-busting medication or surgery to remove clots blocking blood flow in their brain that cause devastating effects like paralysis or even death if left untreated.

Acute emergencies require a prompt response from skilled nurses trained in life-saving techniques who know what actions need to be taken at lightning speed without hesitation regardless of how overwhelming and stressful they might seem at first glance, knowing how critical it can impact someone's life should make you better prepared both mentally & physically.

At the end of this chapter on nursing care for the CNA exam, it's important to remember that caring for patients is not just about following procedures and protocols. It's also about being emotionally present for them.

Nursing can be a stressful and demanding profession, both physically and mentally. However, it's crucial to remember that patients rely on us as their caregivers during some of the most vulnerable moments of their lives.

While it may not always be easy, taking care of ourselves - whether through self-care practices or seeking professional help - can also benefit our patients. By being in good mental health, we're better equipped to handle the emotional needs of those under our care.

In addition to tending to patients' emotional needs, being prepared for acute emergencies is another crucial aspect of nursing care. Regular training and practice drills can help nurses feel more confident and ready for an emergency.

While many technical skills are required to pass the CNA exam and provide quality nursing care, empathy towards patients' emotions and preparedness for unexpected emergencies are equally essential.

Chapter 5

Specialized Care

Introduction to Specialized Care

Are you aware of the duty of CNAs to provide specialized care for patients with physical and psychological problems? As a Certified Nursing Assistant (CNA), you ensure patients take the attention and care they need. This chapter explores the importance of specialized care for these patients and how CNAs can significantly impact their lives.

Importance of specialized care for patients with physical and psychological problems

Providing specialized care for patients with physical and psychological problems is crucial in ensuring their well-being. These individuals require special attention beyond hospital or clinic medical support. Specialized care often involves addressing the patient's physical and emotional needs, which can be challenging.

Patients with physical impairments may face difficulties performing day-to-day activities such as bathing, dressing, or walking. They require specialized care to ensure their safety and comfort while going about their everyday lives. Caregivers must understand these impairments to provide targeted assistance catering to each patient's needs.

On the other hand, individuals with psychological issues like anxiety disorders, depression, or dementia also require specialized care tailored toward improving their mental health and overall quality of life. Such patients need caregivers who are compassionate, empathetic, and emotionally available; someone who understands what they're going through and can provide them with adequate support.

Specialized care helps improve the patient's overall health by preventing complications associated with chronic conditions, such as bedsores or infections caused by poor hygiene practices. It ensures that all aspects of a patient's well-being are considered while providing necessary treatments.

Providing specialized patient care is essential for anyone dealing with physical or psychological problems. Patients deserve top-quality healthcare services catering to every aspect of their well-being - including physical AND emotional support.

Role of the CNA in providing specialized care

It would help if you remember as a Certified Nursing Assistant (CNA), you are essential in providing specialized care to patients with physical and psychological problems. Your duties include:

- Assisting patients with daily activities.
- Monitoring their health status.
- Reporting any changes to the healthcare team.

In providing specialized care, CNAs must have excellent communication skills to interact effectively with patients of different ages, cultures, and backgrounds. It would be best to be compassionate and empathetic toward your patients' needs while maintaining professionalism.

CNAs should understand that each patient has unique care requirements based on their medical history or condition. Therefore, following individualized care plans developed by licensed nurses or other healthcare professionals is crucial.

Beyond typical caregiving tasks like bathing or feeding patients, CNAs must ensure patient safety by implementing fall prevention measures such as bed rails or gait belts. Additionally, they may need to assist in transferring immobile patients using mechanical lifts.

The CNA is indispensable in providing specialized care for physically and psychologically affected individuals. Being attentive listeners who tailor their services based on patients' needs will help improve health outcomes while fostering trust between them and their caregivers.

Physical Problems

Physical impairments can make it difficult for patients to perform even the most basic tasks. Understanding and addressing these issues is crucial in providing specialized care as a CNA. Some common physical problems include mobility limitations, sensory impairments, and chronic pain.

When dealing with patients who have mobility limitations, CNAs should focus on ensuring their safety by providing them with assistive devices such as walkers or wheelchairs. Helping patients maintain proper body positioning when sitting or lying down can prevent further physical complications.

Clear communication becomes essential for those with sensory impairments like hearing or vision impairment. It's important to speak clearly and use visual aids where possible.

Chronic pain can also be debilitating for patients. CNAs should work closely with medical professionals to ensure that any prescribed medication is administered while providing comfort measures such as warm blankets or massages.

By understanding physical impairments and addressing them through specialized care techniques, CNAs play an essential role in improving the quality of life for their patients.

Understanding physical impairments

Being a Certified Nursing Assistant (CNA), you must understand the different physical impairments that patients may suffer from. Physical disabilities can impact a person's ability to perform daily activities, such as eating, dressing, and bathing.

One form of physical impairment is mobility limitations, such as arthritis or multiple sclerosis. CNAS needs to understand the required level of assistance and provide help with movements such as safely transferring from bed to chair.

Another type of disability includes vision and hearing loss, which need extra attention in communication with the patient. As a CNA, you should know to aid them better, clear enunciation while speaking and written instructions should be provided.

The elderly population often suffers from falls due to balance issues or weakened bones. As a CNA providing specialized care for these patients will involve assessing their environment for possible hazards such as loose rugs or cluttered pathways.

Understanding these physical impairments will enable CNAs to provide better care tailored toward individual patient needs. A CNA who takes time to observe each patient's condition creates an enabling atmosphere where both parties feel comfortable enough around one another, leading toward faster recovery periods.

Providing for patient safety

Providing for patient safety is one of the most critical aspects of specialized care that CNAs must be mindful of. Patients with physical impairments are often at a higher risk for falls and other accidents, so CNAS must take steps to prevent these incidents from happening.

One way to ensure patient safety is by keeping the environment free from hazards such as clutter or slippery floors. Checking on patients can also prevent accidents before they happen; CNAs should make sure that patients have everything they need within reach and help them move around if necessary.

Another aspect of providing for patient safety involves properly using equipment like bed rails, lift devices, or wheelchairs. Improper use can cause further harm to vulnerable patients, so CNAS needs to receive thorough training to operate this equipment properly.

Taking proactive measures to ensure patient safety should be a top priority for any CNA working in specialized care. To keep aware of potential hazards and take preventative action, when necessary, CNAs can help to create an environment where patients feel safe, relaxed, and secure during their recovery process.

Care and comfort for patients with physical impairments

Nursing assistants play a crucial role in providing specialized care for patients with physical impairments. Patients with physical limitations require extra care and attention to ensure their safety and comfort.

One of the primary responsibilities of CNAs is assisting or helping patients with their daily activities, such as bathing, dressing, and grooming. For patients who cannot move independently or have limited mobility, the CNA must help them turn and reposition regularly to avoid pressure sores.

Another important aspect of caring for physically impaired patients is ensuring that they are comfortable. The CNA can assist by providing that the patient's bed linens are always clean and dry, adjusting room temperature as needed, and using pillows or cushions for support where necessary.

Patient safety is also essential in specialized care. CNAs must always be alert during transfers from beds to wheelchairs or other devices used by physically impaired individuals.

Nursing assistants are integral in providing specialized care for those with physical limitations. By ensuring patient comfort while prioritizing safety measures through regular turning/repositioning routines and helping transfer movements, CNAs provide a vital service regarding specifically tailored individualized needs one may encounter within their facility setting.

Psychological Problems

In addition to physical impairments, patients may face psychological problems requiring specialized care. These issues can be just as debilitating and disruptive to a patient's life as a physical condition.

As a CNA, it is essential to understand the different psychological problems that patients may experience. It includes mood disorders like depression or anxiety, personality disorders like borderline or narcissistic personality disorder, and psychotic disorders like schizophrenia.

CNAs must provide emotional support and physical care when caring for patients with these conditions. Establishing trust and building rapport with the patient is essential so they feel comfortable opening up about their struggles.

CNAs should also know about medications to treat these conditions and any potential side effects. They should communicate concerning behaviors or changes in the patient's mental state to other healthcare team members.

Providing specialized care for patients with psychological problems requires empathy, patience, and understanding. By recognizing these patients' unique challenges, CNAs can significantly improve their overall well-being.

Understanding psychological problems

Understanding psychological problems is crucial for providing specialized care to patients. As a CNA, you will work with patients with various psychological conditions, including depression, anxiety, and dementia.

Depression is the most common condition that affects many elderly patients. It can lead to sadness, hopelessness, and loss of interest in daily activities. As a caregiver, providing emotional support is crucial by listening and engaging them in activities they enjoy.

Anxiety is another condition that affects many patients. Patients may experience excessive worry or fear, which can distract their ability to perform daily tasks. Caregivers should be patient and understanding while helping patients manage their anxiety through relaxation techniques such as deep breathing exercises.

Dementia is another progressive neurological disorder that impairs cognitive function leading to memory loss, difficulty communicating, and changes in behavior. Understanding how to communicate effectively with these patients requires patience and empathy while utilizing nonverbal cues when necessary.

Understanding psychological conditions requires empathy toward the patient's situation and practical communication skills. By being aware of potential behavioral changes associated with different needs- caregivers are better equipped to provide holistic care for each individual under their watchful eye!

Care of the Dying Patient

Providing emotional support and comfort is paramount when caring for a dying patient. It involves maintaining a compassionate presence, showing empathy, and being attentive to the patient's emotional and psychological needs. Active listening is crucial, offering a non-judgmental ear and allowing patients to express their fears, concerns, and wishes. Creating a peaceful environment is also essential, adjusting lighting and noise levels and providing privacy to foster a calm, soothing atmosphere. Additionally, offering spiritual support is vital, as respecting and facilitating the patient's spiritual or religious practices and providing access to appropriate resources if desired. Assisting with pain management is another critical aspect of care. It includes administering prescribed pain-relieving medications safely and following established protocols. Non-pharmacological interventions, such as positioning, warm/cold packs, massage, and relaxation techniques, can help alleviate pain and discomfort. Collaborating with the healthcare team by effectively communicating observations and patient responses to pain management interventions ensures the patient's comfort and well-being.

Furthermore, facilitating communication between the patient and their loved ones is vital. It involves promoting open dialogue and encouraging the expression of feelings, concerns and wishes related to end-of-life care. Providing information, education, and support to patients and their families helps them make informed decisions during this challenging time.

Postmortem Care

Maintaining the respect and dignity of the deceased is paramount during postmortem care. It involves handling the body with care and treating it with dignity and respect. Healthcare professionals ensure that movements are gentle, and the body is appropriately covered to preserve privacy and maintain dignity. Respecting cultural and religious practices is also essential, and healthcare providers adhere to specific rituals and customs if requested by the deceased's family. Following proper procedures for handling and preparing the body is crucial for maintaining hygiene and preventing the spread of infection. It includes adhering to infection control protocols and using appropriate personal protective equipment (PPE). Properly cleaning and positioning the body is part of the process, ensuring the deceased is prepared for viewing or transportation according to established guidelines. Throughout the postmortem care process, healthcare professionals also support grieving family members, offering comfort and assistance during their loss.

In conclusion, the chapter on specialized care in the CNA exam emphasizes the importance of addressing the unique needs of patients with physical and psychological problems. The primary duty of a Certified Nursing Assistant (CNA) in providing specialized care is vital in ensuring the safety, maintenance, and comfort of these individuals.

When it comes to physical problems, CNAs play a crucial role in providing the safety, care, and comfort of patients with physical impairments. It includes identifying potential hazards and risks, implementing fall prevention strategies, assisting with mobility and transfers, maintaining proper body alignment and positioning, and utilizing assistive devices appropriately.

In terms of psychological problems, CNAs must understand common conditions such as anxiety, depression, and dementia. They provide emotional support and comfort, assist with pain management, facilitate communication between patients and their loved ones, and promote a compassionate presence throughout the care process.

Furthermore, CNAs are involved in caring for dying patients and postmortem care. They offer emotional support and comfort to dying patients, ensuring their dignity and providing pain management as necessary. During postmortem care, CNAs maintain the respect and dignity of the deceased, follow proper procedures for handling and preparing the body, and support grieving family members.

By recognizing and addressing patients' physical and psychological needs, CNAs contribute significantly to their overall well-being and quality of life. CNAs make a valuable difference in the lives of those they serve, providing comfort and support during challenging times through their compassion, knowledge, and specialized care skills.

In preparation for the CNA exam, studying and understanding the principles and best practices related to specialized care for patients with physical and psychological problems is essential. By doing so, CNAs can demonstrate their competency in providing safe and compassionate care, ultimately contributing to the overall quality of healthcare delivery.

Chapter 6

The Role of the CNA (Role of the Nurse AID)

Are you considering a career as a Certified Nursing Assistant (CNA)? Or are you currently working in this role and want to learn more about your responsibilities? Either way, understanding the vital role of a CNA is crucial. CNAs play an essential part in providing quality healthcare services to patients. In this chapter, we'll dive into what CNAs do, why their role is so crucial, and some critical personal and legal considerations for anyone in this field. Let's get started!

What Does a CNA Do?

CNAs are healthcare professionals who work under the supervision of a licensed nurse. They perform various duties to ensure that patients receive adequate care and support. One of their primary responsibilities is to provide basic care, such as bathing, grooming, dressing, and feeding patients.

In addition to these tasks, CNAs help with patient mobility by assisting them in walking or transferring from bed to wheelchair. They monitor and record vital signs like blood pressure, temperature, pulse rate, and respiration. This information helps doctors track changes in a patient's health status.

Moreover, CNAs are responsible for maintaining clean environments for patients. They may be required to change linens, tidy rooms, or sterilize medical equipment.

The role of a CNA is critical in ensuring that patients receive proper attention during their stay at a healthcare facility. From providing personal hygiene assistance to monitoring vital signs and maintaining cleanliness standards - every task contributes to ensuring that each individual receives quality care tailored specifically for them.

The Importance of the CNA Role

The duty of a Certified Nursing Assistant (CNA) is crucial in the healthcare system. CNAs are responsible for providing essential care and support to patients, ensuring their comfort and well-being throughout their treatment.

CNAs perform daily duties, including assisting patients with personal hygiene tasks and grooming. They also help with mobility by transferring patients from beds to wheelchairs or assisting them with walking exercises.

Moreover, CNAs are essential in monitoring the daily tasks of patients, like blood pressure, pulse rate, respiration rate, and body temperature. They keep track of patients' food intake and output levels while maintaining accurate documentation for nurses' reference.

CNAs contribute invaluably to the healthcare system by working closely alongside registered nurses and licensed practical nurses to deliver quality care that promotes health restoration.

The CNA's role is significant in healthcare delivery. Their dedication to service ensures that patients receive adequate attention at all times while promoting faster recovery rates through consistent nursing assistance.

Personal responsibility

As a CNA, you are responsible for the care and well-being of your patients. It includes ensuring their safety, attending to their medical needs, and providing emotional support. With such an important role comes great personal responsibility.

Firstly, it is essential to understand that being a CNA requires professionalism beyond just showing up to work on time. You must always be aware of how your actions can affect those around you and take ownership of any mistakes or oversights.

Another aspect of personal responsibility as a CNA is maintaining open communication with other healthcare professionals involved in the patient's care. It helps to ensure that all individuals involved are aligned with the treatment plans and minimizes the risk of mistakes or misinterpretations.

It is also crucial to stay up-to-date with training requirements and best practices within the field. It will ensure you provide quality care while minimizing risks for yourself and your patients.

Personal responsibility as a CNA means taking ownership of your actions, communicating effectively with others involved in patient care, and staying current with industry standards. By doing so, you can provide exceptional care while promoting safety for all parties involved.

Personal health and safety

As a certified nursing assistant, it is vital to prioritize your health and safety while caring for patients. It means taking precautions to prevent the spread of infectious diseases and avoiding physical strain and injury.

One way to protect yourself from infection is by practicing proper hand hygiene. It includes washing your hands regularly with soap and water or using alcohol-based hand sanitizer when soap is unavailable.

Additionally, wearing appropriate protective equipment such as gloves, masks, and gowns is essential when working with patients with contagious illnesses or infections.

To avoid physical strain on your body, be mindful of how you move patients and use proper lifting techniques. Always ask for assistance if a patient is too heavy or requires more than one person to lift safely.

Don't forget about mental health. Caring for others can take an emotional toll on you as well. Take breaks when needed and seek support from colleagues or supervisors if necessary.

Prioritizing your health and safety will allow you to provide better patient care while preventing workplace burnout or injury.

Disposal of Pointed or Sharp Objects

Handling pointed or sharp objects with extreme care is crucial as a CNA. Disposing of them ensures the safety of both the patient and the healthcare provider.

Before disposing of any sharp object, inspect it for any damages or defects. If there are any issues, dispose of them immediately in an appropriate sharps container.

Sharps containers should be easily accessible in every healthcare facility. They are specifically designed to prevent accidental needle sticks and other injuries that could spread infection or disease.

When using a sharps container, always fill it within its maximum capacity. Properly seal each container before disposing of them in designated areas.

Remember always to follow universal precautions when handling needles and other sharp objects. Use gloves and protective gear whenever necessary to avoid injury from contact with contaminated items.

By taking these steps seriously, CNAs can ensure their health and safety and the well-being of those around them.

Patient rights

As a CNA, it is crucial to understand and respect the rights of patients under your care. Patients have certain legal rights that must be upheld in any healthcare setting.

One of these fundamental patient rights is the right to privacy. Patients have the right to expect that their medical information will keep private and confidential. As a CNA, maintaining confidentiality is essential by not discussing patient information with anyone who doesn't need to know.

Another essential patient right is informed consent. Patients can receive detailed information about their medical treatment before agreeing or refusing treatment options. As a CNA, you should always ensure patients understand their choices and take steps to obtain the necessary consent from them or their designated representatives.

Patients also have the right to refuse treatment and ask for alternative options if they are uncomfortable with specific procedures or medications suggested by healthcare providers. It's vital for CNAs always to listen when communicating with patients so they can address concerns promptly.

In addition, every patient has equal access regardless of age, race, gender identity, etc., which should always respect by caregivers such as CNAs who work diligently towards providing equitable care for all individuals under our responsibility.

Legal Behavior

In summary, the role of a CNA is crucial in providing quality patient care. CNAs are responsible for various tasks such as daily activities, monitoring vital signs, and assisting with medical procedures under the supervision of licensed nursing staff.

It is essential to understand that personal responsibility plays a significant role in being an effective CNA. Maintaining emotional health and safety by wearing protective gear when necessary and disposing of sharp objects appropriately can help prevent accidents.

Furthermore, understanding patient rights ensures that CNAs provide ethical care while respecting their dignity, privacy, and confidentiality.

Following legal behavior guidelines helps ensure that CNAs maintain professional conduct while performing their duties. It includes adhering to state regulations regarding scope-of-practice limitations and avoiding illegal activity while on duty.

By fulfilling these responsibilities effectively as a CNA, one can contribute towards creating an environment where patients receive high-quality healthcare services.

Ethical Behavior

As a CNA, ethical behavior is of utmost importance. It means acting with integrity, honesty, and professionalism at all times. CNAs must follow strict guidelines regarding confidentiality and respecting patients' rights.

One key aspect of ethical behavior is maintaining boundaries. As a healthcare professional, it's important not to cross the line between personal and professional relationships with patients. It can be challenging, as CNAs often form close bonds with those they care for daily.

Another crucial element of ethical behavior is honesty about your CNA capabilities. Knowing your limitations and seeking help from other healthcare team members is essential.

Always remember that you are an advocate for your patients. It means speaking up if you notice unethical or concerning behavior from colleagues or other healthcare professionals involved in patient care. By adhering to high standards of ethical conduct, CNAs have the power to impact their patients' lives positively every day.

Prioritization and time management

As a certified nursing assistant, time management is crucial in ensuring patients receive the care they need throughout their shifts. With multiple patients and tasks, it's essential to prioritize effectively.

One way to prioritize is by assessing each patient's needs and prioritizing based on urgency. For example, if one patient requires medication at a particular time while another needs assistance bathing, you can attend to the drug before moving on to other tasks.

Another effective technique for managing time is delegating tasks appropriately. If other healthcare professionals can assist with specific tasks, don't hesitate to ask for help. It can allow you more time to focus on high-priority tasks that require your attention.

It's also essential to work when caring for patients. By staying organized and focused during each task, you can save valuable minutes throughout your shift which could accumulate into hours over days or weeks.

By prioritizing effectively and practicing efficient time management skills as a CNA, you will ensure that your patients receive the quality care they deserve within their designated timeframe.

Principles of teamwork

Principles of teamwork are essential in the healthcare industry, especially for CNAs. As a CNA, you will work alongside other healthcare professionals to provide quality patient care. Therefore, working as a team is crucial.

One of the principles of teamwork is communication. Good communication ensures that everyone understands their roles and responsibilities. It also helps build team members' trust, leading to better collaboration and effectiveness.

Another principle is respecting diversity within the team. Each member comes from different background and has unique skills and perspectives that contribute to achieving the common goal – providing excellent patient care.

Collaboration is also critical when it comes to teamwork principles. When team members collaborate, they share knowledge, ideas, and resources that help them achieve their goals quickly and efficiently.

Accountability plays a vital role in creating a thriving team environment. Each member should be responsible for their actions or inactions toward patients' outcomes; this means that every mistake or success reflects on each individual's performance and the entire group's output.

Following these principles can create an efficient healthcare environment where individuals feel valued & appreciated while delivering high-quality care services seamlessly with other health professionals despite challenges encountered along the way.

Interpersonal Relations and communication skills in health care

Interpersonal relations and communication skills in healthcare are crucial for the success of a Certified Nursing Assistant (CNA). Effective communication is essential when interacting with patients, their families, doctors, and other healthcare professionals.

As a CNA, you must communicate clearly and effectively with the patient. It includes active listening skills that allow you to understand their needs fully. You should also be able to explain medical procedures or treatments in understandable terms.

In addition to communicating with patients, CNAs must have excellent interpersonal relationships with coworkers. Being part of a team requires good working relationships and cooperation between colleagues. It can help prevent errors from occurring while ensuring the best possible care is provided.

Teamwork is essential to achieve success. CNAS needs to establish trust and respect through effective communication. Good communication can build stronger bonds between colleagues allowing everyone involved in the patient care delivery process to work harmoniously.

As well as verbal communication skillsets like being articulate or having an extensive vocabulary, nonverbal cues such as tone of voice or body language should not be ignored by CNAs since they can make all the difference during interactions within your workplace environment - where body language speaks louder than words sometimes!

Therapeutic communication techniques

Therapeutic communication techniques are essential skills that every Certified Nursing Assistant (CNA) should possess. These techniques enable CNAs to communicate effectively with their patients, understand their needs and respond appropriately. Effective communication is crucial in building trust between the patient and CNA.

Active listening is an effective therapeutic communication technique that helps CNAs understand what their patients say. It involves giving undivided attention to the patient, developing eye contact, nodding when appropriate, and asking relevant questions.

Empathy is another essential therapeutic communication technique that allows CNAs to connect emotionally with their patients. CNAs can provide emotional support and encouragement by understanding patients' feelings about a particular situation or condition.

Open-ended questioning is also an effective therapeutic communication technique CNAs use to encourage patients to express themselves freely without judgment. This type of questioning allows for more detailed responses from the patient while opening up new avenues of conversation.

Paraphrasing is another proper therapeutic technique used by CNAs during conversations with patients. Paraphrasing shows that you have understood what your patient has said; it also enables you to clarify any misunderstandings and ensure effective two-way communication.

Mastering these therapeutic communication techniques will help enhance relationships between CNAs and their patients while improving care delivery outcomes in healthcare services settings.

The role of CNAs in healthcare is crucial as they play a significant part in ensuring the wellness and comfort of patients. They work closely with nurses and other healthcare professionals to ensure their duties perform effectively.

To be an excellent CNA, ethical behavior, good communication skills, teamwork principles, and prioritization are essential traits that one must possess. These qualities are necessary to succeed in this field.

The CNA profession has its challenges, but it can also be rewarding when you see how your efforts have impacted someone's life positively. It takes dedication, hard work, and commitment to succeed as a CNA while always maintaining professionalism.

Therefore, if you're considering pursuing a career as a Certified Nursing Assistant or already working in this field, I hope this article has highlighted some crucial aspects that will help you provide quality patient care while making your job more fulfilling.

Chapter 7

Questions

1. What is the normal range for adult blood pressure?

   a) 80/60 mmHg

   b) 120/80 mmHg

   c) 160/100 mmHg

   d) 200/120 mmHg

2. Which of the following is the proper technique for hand hygiene?

   a) Rinsing hands with water

   b) Using hand sanitizer without water

   c) Wash hands for at least 20 seconds

   d) Using gloves instead of hand hygiene

3. Which of the following vital signs represents the number of breaths per minute?

   a) Pulse rate

   b) Blood pressure

   c) Respiratory rate

   d) Temperature

4. What is the purpose of an incentive spirometer?

    a) To measure oxygen saturation levels

    b) To monitor blood pressure

    c) To promote deep breathing and lung expansion

    d) To administer medication through inhalation

5. Which is an example of proper body mechanics when lifting a heavy object?

    a) Bending at the waist and using only the back muscles

    b) Twisting the body while lifting

    c) Keeping the feet close together

    d) Bending at the knees and using leg muscles to lift

6. What is the recommended duration for performing hand hygiene?

    a) 5 seconds

    b) 10 seconds

    c) 20 seconds

    d) 30 seconds

7. Which of the following is appropriate when assisting a patient with eating?

    a) Feeding the patient rapidly to save time

    b) Offering foods that the patient dislikes

    c) Allowing the patient to choose the food from the provided options

    d) Ignoring the patient's dietary restrictions

8. Which of one is an example of a non-verbal communication technique?

    a) Using clear and concise language

    b) Active listening

    c) Making eye contact and nodding

    d) Offering empathy and support

9. What is the normal range for an adult's oral temperature?

    a) 32-36°C

b) 36-38°C

c) 38-40°C

d) 40-42°C

10. When providing perineal care to a patient, what is the proper technique?

a) Wiping from back to front

b) Using a robust and scented soap

c) Avoiding gloves

d) Cleaning from front to back, using gentle motions

11. What is the most significant organ in the human body?

a) Liver

b) Heart

c) Skin

d) Brain

12. Which one is responsible for carrying oxygen to the body's tissues?

a) Platelets

b) Red blood cells

c) White blood cells

d) Plasma

13. What is the essential function of the kidneys?

a) Regulation of blood sugar levels

b) Production of digestive enzymes

c) Filtration of blood and waste removal

d) Regulation of body temperature

14. Which one is a common symptom of dehydration?

a) Excessive thirst

b) Swollen ankles

c) High blood pressure

d) Elevated body temperature

15. Which one is a risk factor for developing Type 2 diabetes?

    a) Regular exercise

    b) Healthy body weight

    c) High sugar consumption

    d) Non-smoker

16. Which of the best example of a non-communicable disease?

    a) Influenza

    b) Tuberculosis

    c) Hypertension

    d) Hepatitis B

17. Which of the main characteristic of a benign tumor?

    a) Rapid growth and spread to distant organs

    b) Invasive and destructive to surrounding tissues

    c) capable of metastasizing to other parts of the body

    d) Localized and not cancerous

18. Which of the best example of an autoimmune disease?

    a) Asthma

    b) Rheumatoid arthritis

    c) Osteoporosis

    d) Migraine

19. What is the objective of the respiratory system?

    a) Pump blood throughout the body

    b) Filter toxins from the bloodstream

    c) Exchange oxygen and carbon dioxide

    d) Digest and absorb nutrients

20. Which of the one is an infectious disease?

    a) Alzheimer's disease

    b) Parkinson's disease

    c) Influenza

    d) Osteoarthritis

21. Which body system is responsible for transporting oxygen, essential nutrients, hormones, and waste products throughout the body?

    a) Respiratory system

    b) Cardiovascular system

    c) Nervous system

    d) Muscular system

22. Which of the largest organ in the human body?

    a) Liver

    b) Brain

    c) Skin

    d) Kidneys

23. Which of the body systems is responsible for producing movement and generating heat?

    a) Skeletal system

    b) Digestive system

    c) Muscular system

    d) Endocrine system

24. Which body system supports and protects the body, produces blood cells, and stores minerals?

    a) Respiratory system

    b) Lymphatic system

    c) Skeletal system

    d) Urinary system

25. Which one is the essential function of the respiratory system?

    a) Filtration of blood

    b) Regulation of body temperature

    c) Exchange of oxygen and carbon dioxide

    d) Control of voluntary movements

26. Which body system produces and secures hormones to regulate bodily functions?

    a) Endocrine system

    b) Immune system

    c) Digestive system

    d) Reproductive system

27. Which body system breaks down food, absorbs nutrients, and eliminates waste?

    a) Nervous system

    b) Muscular system

    c) Digestive system

    d) Urinary system

28. Which body system filters blood, regulates fluid balance, and produces urine?

    a) Cardiovascular system

    b) Respiratory system

    c) Urinary system

    d) Reproductive system

29. Which of the body systems is responsible for tracing and responding to internal and external stimuli?

    a) Nervous system

    b) Endocrine system

    c) Immune system

    d) Reproductive system

30. Which body system protects the body against pathogens and foreign substances?

    a) Respiratory system

    b) Lymphatic system

    c) Skeletal system

    d) Digestive system

31. What does the prefix "hyper-" mean in medical terminology?

    a) Above or excessive

    b) Below or under

    c) Around or surrounding

    d) Without or absence of

32. Which suffix is commonly used to denote inflammation?

    a) -algia

    b) -itis

    c) -emia

    d) -osis

33. What does the abbreviation "CPR" stand for in healthcare?

    a) Cardiopulmonary resuscitation

    b) Central processing unit

    c) Computerized tomography scan

    d) Cerebrovascular accident

34. Which term refers to the study of tumors or cancer?

    a) Neurology

    b) Oncology

    c) Cardiology

    d) Dermatology

35. What does the prefix "hypo-" mean in medical terminology?

    a) Above or excessive

CNA Study Guide

b) Below or under

c) Around or surrounding

d) Without or absence of

36. Which term refers to the surgical removal of the appendix?

    a) Appendectomy

    b) Hysterectomy

    c) Mastectomy

    d) Tonsillectomy

37. What does the suffix "-ectomy" means in medical terminology?

    a) Inflammation

    b) Surgical removal

    c) Abnormal condition

    d) Enlargement or stretching

38. Which terms refer to studying the nervous system and its disorders?

    a) Gastroenterology

    b) Ophthalmology

    c) Neurology

    d) Orthopedics

39. What does the abbreviation "MRI" stand for in healthcare?

    a) Magnetic resonance imaging

    b) Medical record information

    c) Metabolic rate index

    d) Myocardial infarction

40. Which of the following terms refers to a blood vessel's abnormal enlargement or stretching?

    a) Thrombosis

    b) Embolism

    c) Aneurysm

d) Ischemia

41. What is the primary goal of using proper body mechanics when assisting patient mobility?

   a) Maintaining good posture

   b) Preventing injuries to the caregiver

   c) Ensuring patient comfort

   d) Facilitating efficient movement

42. Which muscle groups should be primarily used when lifting a heavy object or assisting with a patient transfer?

   a) Back muscles

   b) Leg muscles

   c) Arm muscles

   d) Neck muscles

43. What is the proper technique for lifting a patient from a bed to a wheelchair?

   a) Bend at the waist and lift with the back muscles

   b) Keep the back straight and bend the knees

   c) Use only arm strength to lift the patient

   d) Twist the body while lifting

44. When ambulating a patient with a gait belt, where should the caregiver position themselves?

   a) Behind the patient,

   b) In front of the patient,

   c) On the patient's weaker side,

   d) On the patient's stronger side

45. How should the caregiver position their feet when lifting a heavy object or assisting with a patient transfer?

   a) Close together

   b) One foot in front of the other

   c) Feet spread wide apart

d) Standing on tiptoes

46. When a CNA is transferring a patient from a bed to a chair, he should:

   a) Use their body weight to pull the patient,

   b) Keep their back curved while lifting,

   c) Lift the patient quickly to minimize discomfort,

   d) Communicate and coordinate the transfer with the patient.

47. What is the recommended height for the bed or surface when assisting with patient transfers?

   a) Low position, close to the floor

   b) Medium position, around hip level

   c) High position, above shoulder level

   d) It depends on the specific transfer and patient's condition

48. When a CNA uses a mechanical lift to transfer a patient, which of the following is crucial?

   a) Using the lift without any assistance

   b) Moving the patient quickly to save time

   c) Ensuring proper placement and attachment of the lift sling

   d) Performing the transfer without communicating with the patient

49. What is the purpose of utilizing assistive devices, such as walkers or canes, for patient mobility?

   a) To make the patient look more independent

   b) To provide stability and support during ambulation

   c) To speed up the patient's walking pace

   d) To replace the need for caregiver assistance

50. What should the caregiver do if they feel a patient transfer or lift is beyond their physical capabilities?

   a) Proceed with the transfer cautiously

   b) Ask another caregiver to take over

   c) Ignore the discomfort and complete the task

   d) Encourage the patient to try harder

51. Which of the following nutrients is the body's primary source of energy?

   a) Protein

   b) Carbohydrates

   c) Fats

   d) Vitamins

52. How much water should adults drink daily?

   a) 1-2 cups

   b) 4-6 cups

   c) 8-10 cups

   d) 12-14 cups

53. Which of the vitamins is essential for normal vision and immune function?

   a) Vitamin A

   b) Vitamin C

   c) Vitamin D

   d) Vitamin K

54. Which of a good source of dietary fiber?

   a) Meat

   b) Eggs

   c) White bread

   d) Legumes

55. Which nutrient is vital for building and repairing tissues and producing enzymes and hormones?

   a) Carbohydrates

   b) Protein

   c) Fats

   d) Calcium

56. Which of the excellent source of calcium?

   a) Oranges

b) Milk

c) Chicken

d) Nuts

57. Which nutrient is the body's primary source of insulation and protection for organs?

a) Carbohydrates

b) Protein

c) Fats

d) Iron

58. Which is a symptom of dehydration?

a) Increased urination

b) Dry mouth and throat

c) Excessive sweating

d) Rapid heartbeat

59. Which dietary restriction requires the avoidance of gluten-containing foods?

a) Lactose intolerance

b) Celiac disease

c) Hypertension

d) Diabetes mellitus

60. Which of the excellent source of vitamin C?

a) Fish,

b) Citrus fruits,

c) Red meat,

d) Whole grains

61. What are the instructions to prevent the spread of infections?

a) Using hand sanitizer

b) Wearing gloves at all times

c) Covering the mouth and nose when coughing or sneezing

d) Regular handwashing with soap and water

62. When should healthcare workers perform hand hygiene?

a) Only before and after direct patient contact

b) Only when visibly dirty

c) Before and after every patient contact

d) Only when gloves are not available

63. Which of the best example of healthcare-associated infection (HAI)?

a) Common cold

b) Urinary tract infection (UTI)

c) Seasonal flu

d) Food poisoning

64. What is the purpose of wearing personal protective equipment (PPE)?

a) To protect the patient from the healthcare worker

b) To protect the healthcare worker from the patient

c) To make the healthcare worker feel more secure

d) To comply with hospital regulations

65. Which type of PPE should be worn to protect the eyes from splashes, sprays, or droplets?

a) Gloves

b) Gown

c) Mask

d) Goggles or face shield

66. What is the proper order for donning PPE?

a) Gloves, mask, gown

b) Gown, gloves, mask

c) Mask, gown, gloves

d) Gown, mask, gloves

67. How often should disposable gloves be changed during patient care?

   a) Once a day

   b) Every hour

   c) After each patient contact

   d) Only when visibly soiled

68. What is the purpose of standard precautions?

   a) To protect against specific infections

   b) To reduce the risk of bloodborne pathogens

   c) To safely spread all types of infections

   d) To comply with healthcare regulations

69. Which of the example of a bloodborne pathogen?

   a) Influenza virus

   b) Methicillin-resistant Staphylococcus aureus (MRSA)

   c) Tuberculosis (TB) bacteria

   d) Hepatitis B virus

70. What should we do with used disposable sharps, such as needles or lancets?

   a) Place them in regular trash bins

   b) Recycle them if possible

   c) Dispose of them in a puncture-resistant container

   d) Clean and reuse them if they appear undamaged

71. Which of the following is a chronic respiratory disease divided by inflammation and narrowing of the airways?

   a) Asthma

   b) Diabetes

   c) Hypertension

   d) Osteoarthritis

72. Which of the common symptom of diabetes?

    a) Chest pain

    b) Frequent urination

    c) Rash

    d) Vision changes

73. Which is a contagious skin infection caused by bacteria and characterized by redness, swelling, and pus-filled lesions.

    a) Influenza

    b) Meningitis

    c) Cellulitis

    d) Pneumonia

74. Which of the following is a chronic neurodegenerative disorder characterized by tremors, stiffness, and impaired balance and coordination?

    a) Alzheimer's disease

    b) Parkinson's disease

    c) Multiple sclerosis

    d) Rheumatoid arthritis

75. Which viral infection is characterized by a rash, fever, and sore throat?

    a) Influenza

    b) Hepatitis C

    c) Measles

    d) Tuberculosis

76. Which chronic autoimmune disease causes inflammation, pain, and joint stiffness?

    a) Lupus

    b) Fibromyalgia

    c) Gout

    d) Osteoporosis

77. Which bacterial infection primarily affects the lungs and is characterized by persistent cough, fever, and fatigue?

   a) Tuberculosis

   b) Strep throat

   c) Urinary tract infection (UTI)

   d) Malaria

78. Which chronic inflammatory bowel disease that primarily affects the lining of the digestive tract?

   a) Irritable bowel syndrome (IBS)

   b) Diverticulitis

   c) Crohn's disease

   d) Gastritis

79. Which of the following is a chronic skin condition characterized by itchy, inflamed patches of skin?

   a) Psoriasis

   b) Eczema

   c) Rosacea

   d) Hives

80. Which of the following is a common viral respiratory infection characterized by cough, congestion, and sore throat?

   a) Pneumonia

   b) Bronchitis

   c) Influenza

   d) Sinusitis

Chapter 8

Answers & Explanation

1. b) 120/80 mmHg. Explanation: The normal range for adult blood pressure is generally around 120/80 mmHg. This reading indicates a healthy blood pressure level.

2. c) Washing hands with soap and water for at least 20 seconds. Explanation: The proper technique for hand hygiene involves washing hands for at least 20 seconds. This method helps remove dirt, germs, and bacteria effectively.

3. c) Respiratory rate. Explanation: The respiratory rate indicates the number of breaths a person takes per minute. It is an important vital sign to monitor the respiratory function of patients.

4. c) To promote deep breathing and lung expansion. Explanation: An incentive spirometer is a device that encourages patients to take deep breaths and expand their lungs fully. It helps prevent respiratory complications and improve lung function.

5. d) Bending at the knees and using leg muscles to lift. Explanation: Proper body mechanics when lifting a heavy object involves bending at the knees and using the leg muscles rather than straining the back. This technique helps prevent back injuries.

6. c) 20 seconds.Explanation: The recommended duration for hand hygiene, including washing hands or using hand sanitizer, is typically 20 seconds. This duration ensures thorough cleansing of the hands.

7. c) Allowing the patient to choose the food from the options provided. Explanation: When assisting patients with eating, respecting their preferences and autonomy is essential. Allowing the patient to select the food items from the options promotes patient-centered care.

8. c) Making eye contact and nodding. Explanation: Making eye contact and shaking are

non-verbal communication techniques that show attentiveness and understanding. They can help establish rapport and convey empathy.

9. b) 36-38°C. Explanation: The normal range for an adult's oral temperature is generally considered to be around 36-38°C. This range indicates an average body temperature.

10. d) Cleaning from front to back, using gentle motions. Explanation: When providing perineal care, cleaning from front to back using gentle movements is essential. This technique helps prevent the spread of bacteria from the anal area to the urinary and reproductive systems.

11. Answer: c) Skin. Explanation: The skin is the largest organ in the human body. It is a protective barrier, regulates body temperature, and houses various sensory receptors.

12. b) Red blood cells. Explanation: Red blood cells, or erythrocytes, carry oxygen to tissues. They contain hemoglobin, a protein that binds to oxygen molecules.

13. c) Filtration of blood and waste removal. Explanation: The primary function of the kidneys is to filter waste products, excess water, and toxins from the bloodstream, producing urine as a waste product.

14. a) Excessive thirst. Explanation: Excessive thirst is a common symptom of dehydration. When the body lacks sufficient water, it sends signals to the brain to increase fluid intake.

15. c) High sugar consumption. Explanation: High sugar consumption is a risk factor for developing Type 2 diabetes. When you use excessive sugar, this intake can result in insulin resistance and difficulties processing glucose.

16. c) Hypertension. Explanation: Hypertension, or high blood pressure, is an example of a non-communicable disease. Infectious agents do not cause it and cannot be transmitted from person to person.

17. d) Localized and not cancerous. Explanation: A benign tumor is localized and not cancerous. It does not invade surrounding tissues or spread to distant organs like malignant (cancerous) tumors.

18. b) Rheumatoid arthritis. Explanation: Rheumatoid arthritis is an example of an autoimmune disease. Inflammation and pain occur when the body's immune system attacks the joints.

19. c) Exchange oxygen and carbon dioxide. Explanation: The respiratory system is responsible for exchanging oxygen and carbon dioxide. It involves oxygen intake through inhalation and carbon dioxide removal through exhalation.

20. c) Influenza. Explanation: Influenza, famous as the flu, is infectious. A viral infection causes it and can transmit from person to person through respiratory droplets.

21. b) Cardiovascular system. Explanation: The cardiovascular system, consisting of the heart and blood vessels, is responsible for transporting oxygen, necessary nutrients, hormones, and waste products throughout the body via the bloodstream.

22. c) Skin. Explanation: The skin is the largest organ in the human body, serving as a

protective barrier, regulating body temperature, and participating in sensory perception.

23. c) Muscular system. Explanation: The muscular system produces movement and generates heat through muscle contractions. It works in conjunction with the skeletal system.

24. c) Skeletal system. Explanation: The skeletal system provides support and protection to the body, produces blood cells in the bone marrow, and stores minerals such as calcium and phosphorus.

25. c) Exchange of oxygen and carbon dioxide. Explanation: The respiratory system's primary function is to provide oxygen and carbon dioxide through breathing in the body and the environment.

26. a) Endocrine system. Explanation: The endocrine system consists of glands that produce and secrete hormones, which are chemical messengers that regulate various bodily functions and processes.

27. c) Digestive system. Explanation: The digestive system breaks down food through digestion, absorbing nutrients into the bloodstream and eliminating waste products.

28. c) Urinary system. Explanation: The urinary system, which includes the kidneys, ureters, bladder, and urethra, is responsible for filtering blood, regulating fluid balance, and producing urine.

29. a) Nervous system. Explanation: The nervous system detects and responds to internal and external stimuli, coordinates body movements, and maintains homeostasis.

30. b) Lymphatic system. Explanation: The lymphatic system is crucial in defending the body against pathogens and foreign substances and maintaining fluid balance. It includes lymph nodes, lymphatic vessels, and lymphoid organs.

31. a) Above or excessive. Explanation: The prefix "hyper-" in medical terminology indicates above or excessive. For example, hypertension refers to high blood pressure.

32. b) -itis. Explanation: The suffix "-itis" is commonly used in medical terminology to denote inflammation. For instance, appendicitis refers to the inflammation of the appendix.

33. a) Cardiopulmonary resuscitation. Explanation: The abbreviation "CPR" stands for cardiopulmonary resuscitation, an emergency procedure performed to restore the functioning of the heart and lungs.

34. b) Oncology. Explanation: Oncology is the medical branch that studies and treats tumors or cancer.

35. b) Below or under. Explanation: The prefix "hypo-" in medical terminology indicates below or under. For example, hypothyroidism refers to an underactive thyroid gland.

36. a) Appendectomy. Explanation: Appendectomy is the surgical removal of the appendix. It is commonly performed in cases of appendicitis.

37. b) Surgical removal. Explanation: The suffix "-ectomy" in medical terminology indicates

surgical removal. For example, tonsillectomy refers to the surgical removal of the tonsils.

38. c) Neurology. Explanation: Neurology is the branch of medicine that studies and treats the nervous system and its disorders.

39. a) Magnetic resonance imaging. Explanation: The abbreviation "MRI" stands for magnetic resonance imaging, a medical imaging technique used to visualize internal body structures.

40. c) Aneurysm. Explanation: An aneurysm refers to a blood vessel's abnormal enlargement or stretching, usually due to a weakened arterial wall.

41. b) Preventing injuries to the caregiver. Explanation: The primary goal of using proper body mechanics is to prevent injuries to the caregiver while assisting with patient mobility. It involves using correct posture, body alignment, and movement techniques to minimize strain and stress on the body.

42. b) Leg muscles. Explanation: When lifting a heavy object or assisting with a patient transfer, the leg muscles, particularly the muscles in the thighs and buttocks, should be primarily used. It helps to generate power and leverage while minimizing strain on the back.

43. b) Keep the back straight and bend the knees. Explanation: The proper technique for lifting a patient from a bed to a wheelchair is to keep the back straight, bend the knees, and use the leg muscles to generate power. This technique helps to protect the back and maintain stability during the lift.

44. a) Behind the patient. Explanation: When ambulating a patient with a gait belt, the caregiver should position themselves behind them. It allows for better support and control during the ambulation process.

45. c) Feet spread wide apart. Explanation: When preparing to lift a heavy object or assist with a patient transfer, the caregiver should position their feet spread wide apart. It provides a stable support base and helps maintain balance during the lift.

46. d) Communicate and coordinate the transfer with the patient. Explanation: When transferring a patient from a bed to a chair, the CNA needs to communicate and coordinate the transfer with the patient. It ensures the patient feels involved, safe, and informed during the transfer process.

47. b) Medium position, around hip level. Explanation: The recommended height for the bed or surface when assisting with patient transfers is a medium position around the hip level. It minimizes the need for excessive bending or reaching during the transfer.

48. c) Ensuring proper placement and attachment of the lift sling. Explanation: When using a mechanical lift to transfer a patient, it is crucial to ensure appropriate placement and extension of the lift sling. It provides the safety and comfort of the patient during the transfer.

49. b) To provide stability and support during ambulation. Explanation: The purpose of

assistive devices, such as walkers or canes, for patient mobility, is to provide stability and support during ambulation. These devices help improve balance, reduce the risk of falls, and enhance the patient's independence.

50. b) Ask another CNA to take over. Explanation: If a caregiver feels that a patient transfer or lift is beyond their physical capabilities, they must ask another caregiver to take over. Prioritizing safety and avoiding potential injuries to the CNA and the patient is essential.

51. b) Carbohydrates. Explanation: Carbohydrates are the body's primary source of energy. They provide fuel for bodily functions and physical activity.

52. c) 8-10 cups. Explanation: Adults' recommended daily water intake is approximately 8-10 cups or about 64-80 ounces.

53. a) Vitamin A. Explanation: Vitamin A is essential for normal vision, immune function, and the health of the skin and mucous membranes.

54. d) Legumes. Explanation: Legumes, such as beans and lentils, are good sources of dietary fiber. They help promote healthy digestion and can contribute to a feeling of fullness.

55. b) Protein. Explanation: Protein is vital for building and repairing tissues, producing enzymes and hormones, and supporting various bodily functions.

56. b) Milk. Explanation: Milk and other dairy products are good sources of calcium, which is a must for building and maintaining strong bones and teeth.

57. c) Fats. Explanation: Fats are the body's primary insulation and organ protection source. They also need hormone production and nutrient absorption.

58. b) Dry mouth and throat. Explanation: Dry mouth and throat are common symptoms of dehydration. Other symptoms may include thirst, dark-colored urine, fatigue, and dizziness.

59. b) Celiac disease. Explanation: Celiac disease is an autoimmune disorder in which the consumption of Celiac disease is a condition where gluten, which is present in wheat, barley, and rye, can harm the small intestine. As such, individuals with this disease must adhere to a strict gluten-free diet.

60. b) Citrus fruits. Explanation: Citrus fruits, such as oranges, lemons, and grapefruits, are good sources of vitamin C. Vitamin C is essential for immune function, collagen production, and the absorption of iron.

61. d) Regular handwashing with soap and water. Explanation: Regular handwashing with soap and water is a better way to avoid spreading infections. Hand sanitizer should use when soap and water are not available.

62. c) Before and after every patient contact. Explanation: Healthcare workers should perform hand hygiene before and after every patient contact to minimize the risk of spreading infections.

63. b) Urinary tract infection (UTI). Explanation: A urinary tract infection (UTI) acquired in a healthcare setting is an example of a healthcare-associated infection (HAI).

64. b) To protect the healthcare worker from the patient. Explanation: The purpose of wearing personal protective equipment (PPE) is to protect the healthcare worker from exposure to infectious materials and reduce the risk of transmission.

65. d) Goggles or face shields. Explanation: Goggles or a face shield should be worn to protect the eyes from splashes, sprays, or droplets that may contain infectious material.

66. b) Gown, gloves, mask. Explanation: The proper order for donning PPE is a gown first, gloves, and then the mask or respirator.

67. c) After each patient contact. Explanation: Disposable gloves should be changed after each patient contact to prevent cross-contamination between patients.

68. c) To prevent the spread of all types of infections. Explanation: Standard precautions are infection control practices designed to avoid all kinds of diseases in healthcare settings.

69. d) Hepatitis B virus. Explanation: Hepatitis B virus is an example of a bloodborne pathogen. It can use through contact with infected blood or body fluids.

70. c) Dispose of them in a puncture-resistant container. Explanation: Used disposable sharps, such as needles or lancets, should be disposed of in a puncture-resistant container to prevent injuries and potential transmission of infections.

71. a) Asthma. Explanation: Asthma is a chronic respiratory disease divided into inflammation and narrowing of the airways, leading to symptoms like wheezing, shortness of breath, and coughing.

72. b) Frequent urination. Explanation: Frequent urination is a common symptom of diabetes. Other symptoms may include increased thirst, unexplained weight loss, and fatigue.

73. c) Cellulitis. Explanation: Cellulitis is a contagious skin infection caused by bacteria, typically characterized by redness, swelling, and pus-filled lesions.

74. b) Parkinson's disease. Explanation: Parkinson's disease is a chronic neurodegenerative disorder characterized by tremors, stiffness, impaired balance and coordination, and other motor symptoms.

75. c) Measles. Explanation: Measles is a viral infection characterized by a rash, fever, sore throat, and other flu-like symptoms. It is highly contagious.

76. a) Lupus. Explanation: Lupus is a chronic autoimmune disease that causes inflammation, pain, and joint stiffness, along with other symptoms affecting various body systems.

77. a) Tuberculosis. Explanation: Tuberculosis is a bacterial infection that primarily affects the lungs and is characterized by a persistent cough, fever, fatigue, and other respiratory symptoms.

78. c) Crohn's disease. Explanation: Crohn's disease is a long-term inflammatory bowel condition that primarily impacts the digestive tract lining, resulting in stomach pain, diarrhea, and weight loss.

79. b) Eczema. Explanation: Eczema is a chronic skin condition characterized by itchy, inflamed patches of skin. It often occurs in response to specific triggers or allergies.

80. c) Influenza. Explanation: Influenza, famous as the flu, is a common viral respiratory infection characterized by cough, congestion, sore throat, fever, and body aches.

Conclusion

- The Certified Nursing Assistant (CNA) exam is crucial in becoming a certified healthcare professional.
- The candidates must fulfill specific requirements, including completing an approved training program and meeting certain age and educational criteria.
- Registering for the CNA exam involves applying, attaching the required documentation, and paying the fees.
- On exam day, candidates should expect a comprehensive test that assesses their knowledge and skills in various areas of nursing assistance.
- The exam typically consists of a written or computer-based portion and a practical skills evaluation.
- Adequate preparation through studying course materials, practicing skills, and taking practice exams is essential to increase the chances of success.
- After the exam, candidates must wait for the results, usually released within a few weeks.
- Upon passing the CNA exam, individuals can pursue employment opportunities in various healthcare settings, such as hospitals, nursing homes, and home health agencies.
- If a candidate doesn't clear the exam, they may have the opportunity to retake it after a certain waiting period.
- Overall, the CNA exam is a vital milestone for aspiring nursing assistants, providing them with the necessary certification to begin their rewarding careers in healthcare.
- Passing the CNA exam requires diligent preparation and effective test-taking strategies.
- Familiarizing oneself with test tips and techniques can significantly enhance performance on the exam.
- Understanding the structure and content of the exam, along with time management skills, can help you navigate the test efficiently.
- Overcoming test anxiety is crucial for success. Implementing relaxation techniques, maintaining a positive mindset, and utilizing stress-management strategies can help reduce anxiety levels.
- Developing a personalized study strategy is essential. Breaking down the material into

manageable sections, creating a study schedule, and utilizing various resources, such as textbooks, practice exams, and online resources, can optimize learning and retention.

- Candidates must actively engage in the learning process, such as taking thorough notes, participating in study groups, and seeking clarification on challenging topics, which can enhance understanding and memorization.

- Practicing CNA skills regularly, independently and with a partner, is essential for mastering the practical portion of the exam.

- Reviewing and revisiting previously covered material can reinforce knowledge and ensure comprehensive understanding.

- Seeking guidance and support from instructors, mentors, or experienced CNAs can provide valuable insights and advice for exam success.

- A thorough preparation, effective study strategies, and a positive mindset will significantly increase the likelihood of passing the CNA exam and embarking on a successful career in nursing assistance.

- Personal Care: CNAs are crucial in assisting patients with personal care activities such as bathing, oral hygiene, and toileting. These tasks require sensitivity, respect for privacy, and adherence to infection control protocols.

- Dressing and Grooming: Proper dressing and grooming contribute to the well-being and self-esteem of patients. CNAs should assist patients in selecting appropriate attire, maintaining personal hygiene, and ensuring their comfort and dignity.

- Nutrition and Hydration: Adequate nutrition and hydration are vital for maintaining patients' health and promoting recovery. CNAs should help with meal planning, feeding assistance, and monitoring intake to address individual dietary needs.

- Restoration and Maintenance of Health: CNAs support patients in their health restoration and maintenance journey. It involves assisting with exercises, promoting mobility, and facilitating a safe and clean environment to prevent complications.

- Sleep and Rest Needs: Understanding patients' sleep and rest patterns are crucial for promoting their well-being. CNAs should ensure a comfortable sleep environment, respect individual preferences, and assist with relaxation techniques.

- Elimination (Bowel and Bladder): CNAs provide compassionate care in managing patients' elimination needs. It includes assisting with toileting, monitoring bowel and bladder movements, and implementing regularization strategies.

- Mobility, including Bed Mobility: CNAs help patients maintain mobility and independence. They assist with transferring, repositioning, and using mobility aids to prevent muscle weakness and pressure ulcers.

- Circulation and Skin Integrity: CNAs play a role in promoting healthy circulation and preventing skin breakdown. They assist with proper positioning, regular skin assessments, and implementing preventive measures like turning and padding.

- Age-Related Changes: CNAs should understand the physical changes associated with aging. This knowledge helps provide appropriate care, address specific needs, and promote optimal functioning in elderly patients.

- Cognitive and Psychosocial Changes: CNAs must be sensitive to cognitive and psychosocial changes affecting patients' well-being. Providing reassurance, maintaining a familiar routine, and engaging in therapeutic communication are essential skills.

- Care and Use of Assistive Devices: CNAs may assist patients using assistive devices such as walkers, wheelchairs, or hearing aids. Proper training and understanding of these devices ensure patient safety and independence.

- Self-Image, Strength, and Endurance: CNAs support patients in maintaining a positive self-image and promoting strength and endurance through encouragement, motivation, and appropriate exercise programs.

- Psychosocial Needs: CNAs address the psychosocial needs of patients by providing emotional support, fostering social interaction, and promoting a sense of belonging and purpose

- Observation and Reporting Physical Changes: Nursing professionals must keenly observe and report any physical changes in the patient's condition, such as vital signs, skin integrity, and overall appearance. Timely and accurate reporting is crucial for appropriate interventions and treatment.

- Basic Anatomy and Functions of Body Systems: Understanding the fundamentals of human anatomy and various body systems' functions is essential for effective nursing care. This knowledge helps comprehend the interplay between different systems and identify potential issues.

- Characteristics of Body Functions: Nurses should be familiar with the typical attributes of body functions, including respiratory rate, heart rate, blood pressure, pulse check, and temperature. This knowledge enables them to identify deviations from the norm and take appropriate action.

- Observation and Reporting of Behavior Changes: Besides physical changes, nurses should be attentive to patient behavior changes. Documenting alterations in mood, behavior patterns, and cognitive functioning is vital for the early detection of mental health issues or underlying medical conditions.

- Changes in Mental Status (Confusion): Nurses must be skilled in recognizing and responding to changes in mental status, particularly confusion. Implementing appropriate orientation and validation techniques helps to alleviate anxiety, enhance patient safety, and facilitate communication.

- Emotional Stress: Nursing professionals should be aware of the impact of emotional stress on patients' well-being. Providing emotional support, practicing active listening, and employing therapeutic communication techniques can help patients cope with stress and improve their overall experience.

- Mood Status Changes: Monitoring and documenting changes in patients' mood status is essential for identifying potential mental health concerns or variations in response to treatment. If necessary, timely reporting allows for appropriate interventions and referral to mental health professionals.

- Defense Mechanisms: Nurses should know the different defense mechanisms individuals may employ in response to stress or difficult situations. Recognizing these mechanisms assists in providing appropriate support and care.

- Acute Emergency Situations: Nurses must be prepared to handle acute emergencies promptly and efficiently. Acquiring knowledge of emergency protocols, performing life-saving interventions, and remaining calm under pressure are critical aspects of nursing care.

- In conclusion, Chapter 4 has emphasized the significance of observation, reporting, and nursing interventions in patient care's physical and behavioral aspects. CNAs are pivotal in ensuring timely interventions and promoting optimal patient outcomes by actively monitoring patients, recognizing changes, and documenting observations accurately. Additionally, understanding the basic anatomy, body systems, and mental health concepts equips nurses with the knowledge to deliver comprehensive care and holistically address patients' needs.

- Physical Problems: Specialized care is necessary for patients with physical impairments. Nurses should focus on providing safety, maintenance, and comfort for these individuals. It includes addressing mobility challenges, assisting with activities of daily living, and implementing measures to prevent complications like pressure ulcers or falls.

- Providing for the Safety, Care, and Comfort of Patients with Physical Impairments: CNA's role is vital in ensuring the safety and health of patients with physical impairments. It involves creating a conducive environment, utilizing appropriate assistive devices, promoting independence, and offering emotional support.

- Psychological Problems: Patients with psychological problems require specialized care to address their unique needs. Nurses should demonstrate empathy, active listening, and therapeutic communication skills to establish a trusting relationship. Collaborating with mental health professionals and implementing appropriate interventions contribute to better patient outcomes.

- Care of the Dying Patient and Postmortem Care: CNA involves providing vital care for patients nearing the end of their lives and offering support to their families. Nurses should be knowledgeable about pain management, symptom control, and psychosocial support during end-of-life care. Additionally, they should be proficient in postmortem care procedures, ensuring dignity and respect for the deceased while supporting grieving family members.

- In conclusion, Chapter 5 has highlighted the importance of specialized care for patients with physical and psychological needs and end-of-life care. By addressing these patients' unique challenges, nurses can enhance their quality of life, promote their well-being, and support their families during difficult times. Providing safe, compassionate, and holistic care is at the core of specialized nursing, empowering patients to maintain their dignity and optimizing their overall experience within the healthcare system.

- Personal Responsibility: CNAs provide quality care, maintain professional boundaries, and adhere to ethical standards. They should prioritize patient safety and advocate for their well-being.

- Personal Health and Safety: CNAs must prioritize their health and safety by following infection control protocols, using personal protective equipment (PPE), and practicing proper body mechanics to prevent injuries.

- Disposal of Pointed or Sharp Objects: Proper disposal of sharp objects, such as needles or scalpels, is essential for preventing injuries and maintaining a safe environment. CNAs should follow the facility's guidelines for disposal.

- Patient Rights: CNAs should respect and uphold patients' rights, including privacy, dignity, informed consent, and autonomy. They should ensure that patients know their rights and provide support when needed.

- Legal Behavior: CNAs must understand and adhere to legal requirements and regulations related to their role. It includes confidentiality, documenting accurately, and reporting incidents or concerns according to legal protocols.

- Ethical Behavior: CNAs should uphold ethical principles, such as honesty, integrity, and respect for cultural diversity. They should demonstrate empathy, maintain professional boundaries, and make ethical decisions when faced with challenging situations.

- Prioritization and Time Management: CNAs should possess strong prioritization and time management skills to handle multiple tasks and provide timely care to patients effectively. It involves identifying urgent needs, organizing workloads, and collaborating with the healthcare team.

- Principles of Teamwork: CNAs play a vital role in the healthcare team. They should actively participate in interdisciplinary collaboration, communicate effectively, and contribute to a supportive and respectful team environment.

- Interpersonal Relations and Communication Skills in Healthcare: CNAs should develop solid interpersonal relations and practical communication skills to establish rapport with patients, families, and colleagues. It includes active listening, empathy, and adapting communication styles to meet individual needs.

- Therapeutic Communication Techniques: CNAs should utilize therapeutic communication techniques to promote a positive patient experience. It involves using open-ended questions, reflective listening, and emotional support during challenging situations.

- In conclusion, Chapter 6 has emphasized the crucial role of the CNA in providing responsible, ethical, and compassionate care. By understanding their responsibilities, upholding patient rights, adhering to legal and ethical standards, and effectively communicating within the healthcare team, CNAs contribute to the overall well-being and satisfaction of patients. Their commitment to personal health and safety ensures a secure work environment for themselves and others. CNAs significantly impact the healthcare field through their professionalism and dedication and play a vital role in delivering quality patient care.

Made in the USA
Middletown, DE
27 September 2023

39546302R00064